ADVANCE PRAISE FOR *THE MENOPAUSE BRAIN*

"In a society that often downplays the significance of menopause and its impact on women's lives, Dr. Mosconi's book serves as a rallying cry for embracing this transformative period with knowledge and empowerment. Her insights remind me of the importance of fostering a sense of community and support among women, a sentiment I hold dear in my own work."

Dr Mary Claire Haver, bestselling author of *The Galveston Diet*

"Every woman should know that menopause is more than just mood and hot flashes; it can profoundly impact brain health and function. Dr. Lisa Mosconi stands as a foremost expert on the menopause brain. This outstanding new book is a must-read, and I wholeheartedly recommend it."

Naomi Watts

"Written and referenced with care but phrased in a lighthearted, easy-to-understand style, this book is highly recommended for women who want to actively participate in preserving their brain's health as they approach and progress through perimenopause and menopause."

Dr Avrum Bluming, co-author of *Estrogen Matters*

"In *The Menopause Brain*, Dr. Lisa Mosconi expertly guides us so that we do not feel alone in this journey, providing us with hope and achievable, empowering solutions drawn from her pioneering research, holistic training, and personal experience."

Tamsen Fadal, author of *The New Single*

"When it comes to menopause, it feels as if we have no information, misinformation, or what's out there is too chaotic and conflicting to make sense. Enter Lisa Mosconi. Hallelujah and thank you! Written with a neuroscientist's mind and a woman's heart, this book is packed with evidence-based, empowering information on all things menopause. For every woman living any phase of menopause, this is your required reading."

Lisa Genova, bestselling author of *Still Alice*

*

Dr Lisa Mosconi is the associate director of the Alzheimer's Prevention Clinic at Weill Cornell Medical College/New York-Presbyterian Hospital, where she was recruited as an associate professor of Neuroscience in Neurology. She also is an adjunct faculty member in the Department of Psychiatry at NYU School of Medicine, in the Department of Nutrition at NYU Steinhardt School of Nutrition and Public Health, and in the Departments of Neurology and Nuclear Medicine at the University of Florence. Dr Mosconi holds a dual PhD degree in Neuroscience and Nuclear Medicine from the University of Florence, Italy, and is a board-certified integrative nutritionist and holistic healthcare practitioner.

The
Menopause
Brain

THE NEW SCIENCE EMPOWERING
WOMEN TO NAVIGATE MIDLIFE WITH
KNOWLEDGE AND CONFIDENCE

DR LISA MOSCONI

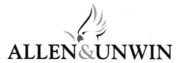

ALLEN&UNWIN

First published in Great Britain in 2024 by Allen & Unwin
First published in the United States in 2024 by Avery, an imprint of
Penguin Random House LLC

Allen & Unwin
c/o Atlantic Books
Ormond House
26–27 Boswell Street
London WC1N 3JZ
Phone: 020 7269 1610
www.atlantic-books.co.uk

A CIP catalogue record for this book is available from the British Library.

Designed by Neuwirth & Associates

Trade paperback ISBN 978 1 83895 749 0
E-book ISBN 978 1 83895 750 6

Printed and bound by CPI (UK) Ltd, Croydon CR0 4YY

10 9 8 7 6 5 4 3 2 1

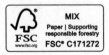

FSC
www.fsc.org
MIX
Paper | Supporting
responsible forestry
FSC® C171272

To all women—our ancestors, our descendants,

and all of you blazing the trail with me as we speak.

CONTENTS

FOREWORD

I AM SO HAPPY that you picked up *The Menopause Brain*. Good for you. You just did yourself and your brain a huge favor! Now that you have this book, you will not have to navigate perimenopause, menopause, or even your postmenopausal life alone. You now have at your fingertips the most up-to-date information about what is happening to your brain and your body—and why. What a gift!

This book is crucial because every woman, if she lives long enough, will go through menopause at some point in her life. And every woman will wonder why, in addition to losing her period and fertility, she may be experiencing sudden heart palpitations, anxiety, depression, lack of concentration, hot flashes, night sweats, mood swings, and sleep disturbances. The list of symptoms is long and varied. Menopause is a function of the brain that plays havoc with a woman's body and her outlook on life. Indeed, all of these erratic emotions and symptoms can make a woman feel crazy if she is not reassured that they are normal. This book will do exactly that.

I wish this book had been around when I was going through perimenopause and menopause because for millions of women like me, when *The Big M*, as I call it, came knocking, we were given little information to guide us forward. So women of my generation felt unseen and unheard by healthcare professionals who weren't educated in this space and didn't have the research to help guide us through the confusing, often chaotic symptoms we were experiencing. Instead, we weathered the turbulence, while living in a culture that intimated women at midlife were prone to going crazy. This book is testimony to progress.

A few years ago, I was honored to write the foreword to Lisa's book *The XX Brain*, and now I am thrilled to write the foreword to this book as well. In *The Menopause Brain*, you have the most current science and the best practical guidance available, and it comes from a researcher who is not only an innovative and visionary thinker but someone I now consider a friend for life.

I first met Lisa in 2017, when I was looking for research to help answer the questions of why women are twice as likely to develop Alzheimer's as men, and why women of color are at even higher risk for the disease. Finding almost no research available motivated me to start my nonprofit organization, the Women's Alzheimer's Movement (WAM), and it has driven my quest ever since to learn about women's brains throughout the lifespan. Meeting Lisa along this journey was a game changer. She was one of the first scientists to show the impact of menopause on a woman's brain at midlife, and to discuss the brain's response to menopause in general. Lisa had just published the first study showing that women's brains become more vulnerable to Alzheimer's in the years before and after menopause. She was among the first researchers who not only described how a woman's brain changes physically and shrinks during menopause, but developed the technology and research to show the process in action. Thanks to Lisa and other like-minded scientists dissatisfied with the lack of research on women's brain health, a movement began that aimed to study the unique impact of sex hormones such as estrogen on women's health. I was delighted to help fund some of that research through the WAM Research Grants, which are awarded to scientists looking at the role of gender as a risk factor for Alzheimer's.

It's a sad fact that despite the prevalence of menopause symptoms and its potentially serious consequences on long-term health, research into menopause has historically been underfunded and overlooked, right alongside women's health in general. For Black women in particular, the health consequences of this oversight are even more dire, and the road through menopause often longer and harder. There is no excuse for ignorance.

My mission now is to make up for lost time, for the neglect in funding that has led to a historic gap in our understanding of women's health. It's why in 2022 we joined forces with one of the world's top-rated healthcare systems to become WAM at Cleveland Clinic. I'm proud to say WAM remains the preeminent organization for women and Alzheimer's, made all the stronger by now having partners leading the field in medical research and excelling at delivering the best clinical care available. In 2020 we made history together when we opened the first Alzheimer's Prevention Center designed just for women at the Lou Ruvo Center for Brain Health in Las Vegas. Now we are working on a shared mission to make Cleveland Clinic a premier holistic center for women's healthcare where every patient feels seen and heard.

My focus is on continuing to support all those around the world who, like Lisa, are researching what is happening to women's brains during midlife, while also ensuring that women everywhere get the valuable information they need to take control of their health during these critical decades. And it's not just women who need to have this information but their doctors, friends, and families as well. This book is a guide for us all, and I hope it is studied by those teaching medicine and those practicing it. I encourage women to remember that they can make a difference to their own health. I hope they will visit their healthcare providers with this book and its research in hand, and together formulate a plan that will deliver them the best medical care they need and deserve to set them up for lifelong health.

So empower yourself with this knowledge, share it with women you meet along the journey. Become what I call an "architect of change"—someone who brings about the change they want to see in the world. Your brain is your biggest asset. Care for it well so it may last a lifetime. I promise it will be the best investment you can make in your future health.

—*Maria Shriver*

PART 1

THE BIG M

1

You Are Not Crazy

"AM I LOSING MY MIND?"

Between the ages of thirty and sixty, many women will wake up one morning and wonder what hit them. Whether it's uncontrollable sweating or a barrage of brain fog and anxiety, any one of us can be confronted with an onslaught of peculiar changes sudden enough to, quite literally, make her head spin.

It might be a sense of disorientation, where you find yourself doing increasingly absent-minded things, like entering a room only to wonder what made you go there in the first place. Belongings may be misplaced, with milk cartons finding their way into cabinets and cereal boxes ending up in the fridge. Communication can also become a challenge. Moments of sheer panic may arise as you struggle to come up with that word on the tip of your tongue or draw a blank on something you just said, losing your train of thought. Emotions, too, can be all over the place, as if a heavy darkness is causing you to weep for no clear reason—only to be replaced a moment later by waves of irritability or even anger. And just when you hoped a good night's sleep might resolve these issues, sleep becomes elusive. Like a fickle ghost, it visits sporadically throughout the night, or may not appear at all. With the rapid-fire onset and the intensity of these unexpected changes, it's no wonder many feel as if their own bodies are betraying them, throwing any woman into a tailspin of questioning herself, her health, and even her sanity.

Perhaps you don't recognize any of these symptoms—yet. Most likely, though, you've heard about them before. From girlfriends, from your mother, from googling late at night when you can't sleep . . . again.

We now have a name for it: menopause brain.

More often than not, the answer to the phenomena so many women experience in midlife is nothing more, but also *nothing less,* than menopause.

Menopause is one of the best-kept secrets in our society. Not only has there been no proper education or culture of support around this rite of passage common to all women, but often, menopause isn't even discussed within families. What's noteworthy is that even when there is some information or wisdom that's shared, it's generally not centered around the most prominent aspects of the transition—namely, how menopause impacts *the brain.*

As a society, insofar as we have understood menopause at all, it's generally only half of what it's all about—the half that pertains to our reproductive organs. Most people are aware that menopause marks the end of a woman's menstrual cycle and, therefore, her ability to bear children. But when the ovaries close up shop, the process has far broader and deeper effects than those associated with fertility. Far from the spotlight, menopause impacts the brain just as much as it impacts the ovaries—directly and powerfully, and in ways we are only beginning to gather real data about.

What we do know is that all these baffling symptoms—the heat surges, the feelings of anxiety and depression, the sleepless nights, the clouded thoughts, the memory lapses—are, in fact, symptoms of menopause. The real kicker, however, is that they don't originate in the ovaries at all. They are initiated by another organ entirely: *the brain.* These are, in fact, *neurological* symptoms that come from the ways that menopause changes the brain. As much as your ovaries have their role in this process, it's your brain that's at the wheel.

Does that make your worst fear real? Are you truly losing your mind?

Not at all. I am here to reassure you that you are *not* going crazy. Most important to note: you are not alone in this, and you are going to be okay. While menopause does indeed impact the brain, that doesn't mean the problems we experience are "all in our head." Just the opposite.

THE HIDDEN SCALE AND IMPACT OF MENOPAUSE

In our youth-obsessed culture, where it's not outright dismissed, menopause is either dreaded or derided. Not only is there no acknowledgment of menopause as a noteworthy landmark in a woman's life, but as it is historically perceived in the extreme negative, menopause comes with the stigmas associated with ageism, the demise of one's vitality, and even the end of our identity as women. Mostly, however, menopause is framed in silence, sometimes even secrecy. Generations of women have suffered under misinformation, shame, and helplessness. Many remain reluctant to discuss their symptoms for fear of being judged, or strive to hide them. Most don't even realize that what they're experiencing has anything to do with menopause in the first place.

All this confusion isn't just unfair. It constitutes a significant public health problem, with far-reaching consequences. Let's look at the numbers:

- Women are half of the population.
- All women go through menopause.
- Women of menopausal age are by far the largest growing demographic group. By 2030, 1 billion women worldwide will have entered or will be about to enter menopause.
- Most women spend about *40 percent of their lives* in menopause.

- All women, menopausal or not, possess an organ that has been largely ignored: the brain.
- Over three-quarters of all women develop *brain symptoms* during menopause.

Out of sheer numbers alone, menopause should be a major sociocultural event and the subject of extensive investigation and deep knowledge. Instead, whether we remain focused on the unpleasant symptoms or psyched out by the perceived lessening of our female powers, the current perception of what menopause means is fixated on the many pitfalls of this life event. Meanwhile, from a scientific and a medical perspective, it's a discipline without a name.

The Problem of Western Medical Frameworks

Thanks to how genuinely uninformed we are about menopause, too many women are caught completely off guard, feeling betrayed by their body *and* their brain—not to mention their doctors, too. While hot flashes are generally recognized as a "side effect" of menopause, most doctors simply won't make the connection between menopause and its other symptoms such as anxiety, insomnia, depression, or brain fog. This is especially the case for women under fifty, who are typically sent home with a prescription for antidepressants, their concerns dismissed as a by-product of their psychology, a sort of female existential crisis. Why is that?

Western medicine is well known for its siloed, non-holistic frameworks, in which the human body is evaluated in terms of its individual components. For example, people with eye problems go to an eye doctor, and those with heart problems go to a cardiologist even if the heart problems led to the eye problems. As a result of this extreme specialization, menopause has been pigeonholed as "an issue with the ovaries" and consigned to ob-gyn territory. Anyone who's been there, however, knows that ob-gyns don't do brains. Educated like every other doctor to specialize in specific body parts—in this case, the reproductive system—they aren't trained to diagnose or manage brain symptoms in the first place. But also, many ob-gyns are not trained to manage menopause at all. Today, fewer than one in five ob-gyn residents receive formal training in menopause medicine, which often consists of a mere few hours in total. Perhaps unsurprisingly, 75 percent of women who seek care for menopausal symptoms end up not receiving treatment.

On the other hand, brain doctors—neurologists and psychiatrists, among others—don't handle menopause, either. Given these divided frameworks, it's no surprise that the effects of menopause on brain health have been neglected, leaving these issues to fall into the cracks between rigidly defined medical disciplines.

Here's where brain scientists come in handy. I am one of them, holding a somewhat unusual PhD in neuroscience (the study of how the brain works) and nuclear medicine (a branch of radiology that uses imaging techniques to examine the brain). But what really sets my work apart is that I have made it my life's work to study and support *women's* brains. Specifically, I am an associate professor of neuroscience in neurology and radiology at Weill Cornell Medicine in New York City, where I apply this background at the intersection of all these disciplines and women's health. To this aim, in 2017, I launched the Women's Brain Initiative, a clinical research program entirely and unapologetically dedicated to understanding how brain health plays out differently in women than in men. All day every day, my team studies women's brains—how they work, what makes them uniquely powerful, what makes them uniquely vulnerable. At the same time, I am the director of the entire Alzheimer's Prevention Program at Weill Cornell Medicine/NewYork-Presbyterian, which allows me to integrate my research on women's brains with the clinical practice of evaluating and supporting cognitive and mental health for the long run.

Years of research have made clear to me that caring for the health of the female brain requires a careful understanding of how it shifts and changes in response to our hormones, especially during menopause. So one of the very first things I did after launching these programs was to pick up the phone and call the ob-gyn department. From that day on, we've been collaborating with some of the best menopause specialists around, as well as top-tier ob-gyn surgeons and oncologists. Together we set out to answer the question we didn't see enough professionals exploring: *How does menopause impact the brain?*

THE BRAIN ON MENOPAUSE

When I started studying menopause, I quickly realized two important facts. First, very few brain studies looked at menopause at all. Second, the few that did were focused on women who were well past menopause, often in their sixties and seventies. In other words, menopause has been studied in terms of its impact on the brain *after* the fact— more like a product than a process.

My team and I have focused instead on what leads to those outcomes, up to and through menopause. To give you a sense of how dire the situation looked when we started, there wasn't a single study that examined women's brains before and after menopause. So we rolled up our sleeves, turned on the brain scanner, and set out to explore this new frontier. As of today, we've made significant progress in demonstrating that women's brains age differently from men's brains, and that menopause plays a key role here. In fact, our

Figure 1. Brain scans before and after menopause

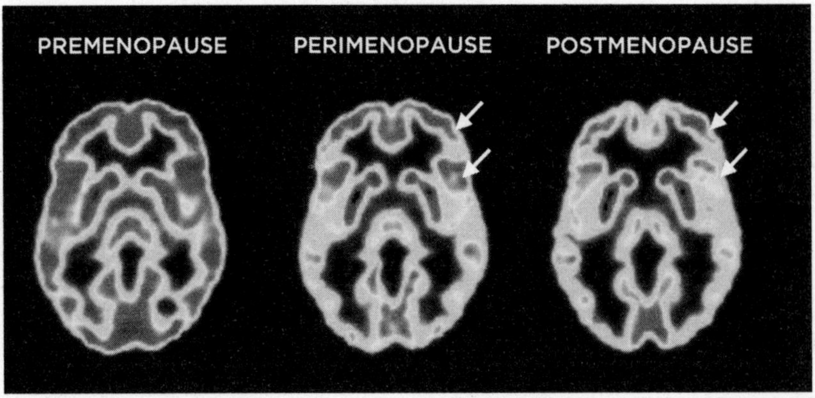

studies have shown that menopause is a *neurologically active process* that impacts the brain in fairly unique ways.

To give you a sense of this, what you see on the previous page is a type of brain scan generated by a functional imaging technique called positron emission tomography, or PET, that measures brain energy levels. Brighter colors indicate high brain-energy levels, while the darker patches indicate a lower energy turnover. (For full-color imagery, see my website: https://www.lisamosconi.com/projects.)

The image to the left shows a high-energy brain. It is a perfect example of what you want your brain to look like when you're in your forties—vivid and bright. This brain belongs to a woman who was forty-three years old when scanned for the first time. Back then, she had a regular cycle and no symptoms of menopause.

Now look at the scan labeled *postmenopause*. That's the same brain just eight years later, shortly after the woman had gone through menopause. Do you notice how this scan looks darker overall than the first? That change in luminosity reflects a 30 percent drop in brain energy.

This finding was far from being an isolated case; many women enrolled in our research program exhibit similar changes, whereas men of the same age do not. So what you see here are intense shifts that seem specific to the female brain going through menopause. While these changes can account for feeling worn out or simply out of sorts (as many can attest to, menopause fatigue is nothing to sneeze at), they sink more than your energy. They can also impact your body temperature, mood, sleep, stress, and cognitive performance. And guess what? Most women can *feel* these changes. When there are marked biological changes at play, resulting in actual modifications of the brain's very chemistry, one can't help but notice them.

The aforementioned study was only the tip of the iceberg. Over time, our investigations yielded a treasure trove of data, demonstrating that it's not just brain energy that changes during menopause but that the brain's structure, regional connectivity, and overall chemistry are also impacted. All of this can make for a profoundly mind-blowing, mind-body experience. Perhaps less obvious without a brain scanner is that these changes don't occur after menopause—they start before it, during perimenopause. Perimenopause is the warm-up act to menopause in which you start skipping periods and symptoms like hot flashes tend to make their first appearance. Our research shows that's exactly when the brain is going through the most profound changes, too. The best way I can explain this phenomenon is that the menopause brain is in a state of adjustment, even remodeling, like a machine that once ran on gas and is now switching to electricity, challenged to find work-arounds. But mostly, these findings are scientific evidence of what scores of women have been saying all along: *menopause changes your brain*. So if you've ever been told that your symptoms are just stress-related or "part of being a woman," here's the proof that all you've been experiencing is scientifically valid and viable. The brain is at the crux of the matter, not your imagination.

How Science Can Help

Over the years, I've spoken to countless women in various states of distress due to menopause, especially as related to their brain symptoms (whether they could articulate these or not). Many have told me that one of their steepest challenges was finding information they could not only readily consume but also trust. Hearing and listening to their need for knowledge and support made me realize that every woman deserves accurate and thorough information about menopause. Peer-reviewed science ensures that the ideas are valid, but academic journals are not an efficient way to provide this information to the hundreds of millions of women in the real world.

The Menopause Brain grows out of my commitment to empowering women with the information they need to experience menopause with knowledge and confidence. Understanding what's happening inside your body and brain before, during, and after menopause is crucial to understanding *yourself* before, during, and after menopause. It is just as crucial to take charge of your changing healthcare needs and reclaim your agency during this important life transition.

Thus far, menopause has been painted as an ill-fated, flat-out scary roadblock ahead, coming for us one by one. Most of what's been written about menopause, from the scientific literature to online sources, focuses on coping or dealing with it, if not even rebelling against it. The vast majority of research on the topic has also been focused on what can go wrong with menopause and how you can "fix it." "What's wrong with that?" you may ask. Underlying this approach is the assumption that we can't hope for better than surviving menopause. By treating this life event strictly in a biological context, Western medicine has emphasized its downsides and minimized its significance. But when you look at menopause from an integrative perspective, there is much more at play. In reality, the hormonal changes that provoke menopause and its symptoms are simultaneously fostering the development of new and intriguing neurological and mental skills—ones our society blatantly chooses to ignore. The hidden powers of the mind on menopause are the highlights that never make the headlines, powers that all women should be aware of. Such awareness leads to new means of navigating menopause, and ultimately womanhood itself.

To this end, the book is divided into four parts:

Part 1, "The Big M," provides the foundational elements needed to understand what menopause is and isn't, from a clinical perspective; how it impacts the brain; and how we fail to recognize this crucial connection.

Part 2, "The Brain-Hormone Connection," discusses the role of hormones for brain health and how this interplay is critical in understanding menopause. Here, we take a deep dive into understanding how menopause operates within the body and brain, which is not just about deciphering the "what" but also the "why" of menopause, placing it within a broader context. To do so, we will examine what I call the Three P's: puberty, pregnancy, and perimenopause. These are all pivotal times during which our brains, hormones, and the give-and-take between them change dramatically. Knowledge of the similarities between the Three P's is key to recontextualizing menopause as a natural stage in a woman's life—a moment that, just like the others, can provoke vulnerability as well as resilience and positive change. However, if your immediate interest lies in finding solutions and seeking ways to feel better, feel free to skip to part 3, where we focus on practical strategies and guidance. Part 2 will be there for you whenever you're ready!

Part 3, "Hormonal and Nonhormonal Therapies," is a deep dive into hormone replacement therapy, as well as other hormonal and non-hormonal options for menopause care. We will then review anti-estrogen therapy for breast cancer and ovarian cancer, and the effects of "chemo brain." Finally, while throughout the book I use the term "women" to refer to individuals born with a so-called female reproductive system (breasts and ovaries), not all people who go through menopause identify as women and not all people who identify as women go through menopause. In recognition of the diverse experiences and identities within the context of menopause, we will discuss gender-affirming therapy for transgender individuals, which includes methods to suppress estrogen production.

Part 4, "Lifestyle and Integrative Health," discusses key validated lifestyle and behavioral practices designed to address the symptoms of menopause without prescription medications, while also supporting cognitive and emotional health. Although you might feel like your brain is all over the place, you do have control over your lifestyle, environment, and mindset—all of which can impact your experience of menopause in return. There is a way to be empowered by embracing and caring for menopause; as we do, a wealth of new possibilities is made evident.

Ultimately, this book is a love letter to womanhood and a rallying cry for all women to embrace menopause without fear or embarrassment. It's the foundation to celebrate our own signature brand of brainpower, to appreciate the intelligent adaptations our bodies and brains make over the course of a lifetime, and to enjoy our journey to optimal lifelong health. I hope the information contained in this book will spur many a discussion, not only about the multifaceted topic of menopause but also about the way in which we have dismissed and marginalized various important parts of our population at large. This is crucial not only to shift the conversation about menopause but also to reinvigorate the voice of the "forgotten gender"—individually, and as half the world.

2

Busting the Bias Against Women and Menopause

SEXISM AND NEURO-SEXISM

This book is a neuroscientist's take on the ups and downs of menopause. Before we reveal the future of the field, however, it's useful (albeit a bit dismaying) to review the cultural and clinical perspectives on menopause to date. I warn you that retracing some key sociohistorical steps on the topic might leave you feeling gloomy at first. After all, the combo of culture and conventional medicine is the reason we equate menopause with "ovarian failure," "ovarian dysfunction," "estrogen depletion," and another slew of negative outcomes. But stick with me; I promise that if we draw from modern science, there's a very different and more balanced story to tell.

From a cultural perspective, however, the outlook is unequivocally dim. If we dig a little deeper, it's clear that many of the demeaning stereotypes around menopause originate from a broader negative understanding of women* as the "weaker sex." If we start with the

---

* Throughout the book, for the sake of simplicity and based on the long-standing biological definition of the female sex, I use the term "women" to refer to individuals who were born with two XX chromosomes and possess a female reproductive system (including breasts and ovaries). However, there are individuals who fit within this biological framework but do not identify as women, and there are also individuals who

age-old sense that women are physically more fragile than men, this reference is also applied to our brains and intellect in the form of what we now call *neuro-sexism*—the myth that women's brains are inferior to men's brains. So before we can even address the complexity of medical frameworks for menopause, we need to address the complexity of the same frameworks for women as a whole.

However astoundingly flawed the doctrine of female inferiority may be, it's nothing short of the backbone of modern science. According to Charles Darwin, the father of modern biology, "a man attains a higher eminence, in whatever he takes up, than can women—whether requiring deep thought, reason, or imagination, or merely the use of the senses and hands." This theory gathered momentum and proliferated unchallenged throughout the nineteenth century, when male scientists made an "impressive discovery." They realized not only that women's heads were anatomically smaller than men's but that women's brains weighed less than men's as well. This was an era in which the biological premise that "bigger is better" reigned supreme. Therefore, a woman's slender brain was conveniently interpreted as a sign of lack of intelligence and mental inferiority. The pundits of the day were quick to correlate that with a lack of aptitude for a variety of tasks. For example, George J. Romanes, a leading evolutionary biologist and physiologist of the time, went on to say this: "Seeing that the average brain-weight of women is about five ounces less than that of men, on merely anatomical ground we should be prepared to expect a marked inferiority of intellectual power in the former." These assumptions were by no means unique, as most intellectuals back then were perfectly comfortable embracing an interpretation that suited the status quo. Those "missing five ounces" of women's brains were thus used to justify the difference in the social status between men and women,

---

were not born with these characteristics but do identify as women or as female. The biological response discussed in this chapter is independent of gender identity and rooted in physiology. Chapter 12 is focused on discussing the diverse experiences of individuals beyond the traditional biological definitions.

cementing the denial of women's access to higher education or to other rights that might have rendered them independent.

I'm going to go out on a limb here and guess that the following goes without saying: the fact that, on average, men's bodies are larger and heavier than women's might have made the observation that their heads were more or less made to match a no-brainer (pun intended). If one has a bigger body, the skull and the brain within should be bigger as well. In fact, once head size is taken into account, the fabled brain-weight difference disappears into the thin air whence it came.

Just the same, for centuries, women's brains continued to be weighed and found wanting, keeping women out of universities and prestigious jobs. Eventually, female scientists and human rights activists joined forces to denounce how such biased interpretations were nothing more than political weaponry subverting women's efforts to attain equity and equality. Thanks to their efforts, the brain-weight intelligence theory was fully debunked in the early twentieth century. The later advent of brain imaging fostered further progress in dispelling many of the base assumptions behind neuro-sexism, leveling the playing field once and for all.

Or has it?

Today, while overtly sexist statements no longer have a place within the scientific community, many argue that neuro-sexism is still alive and kicking. The thing is, in many respects women's brains do differ from men's. We'll talk more about this in just a moment. For now, I want to point out that disparities between the genders are too seldom used to modernize medical care, and far too often used to reinforce demeaning gender stereotypes instead. Consciously or not, we are coerced into gender roles from birth, further fed by pop science claims about how our "Venus/Mars" behaviors differ due to our brains. It may start with the age-old tradition of accessorizing our infants in pink and blue, but it ends with the propagation of rigid, derogatory biases that relentlessly cast women as the lesser gender.

As it now stands, we face a triple challenge: sexism, ageism, and *menopause-ism*. From the moment we are born, the message from our society is that we are lesser as women, if for no other reason than the fact that men are bigger and stronger. But these baseline beliefs proliferate in ways both subtle and not as we traverse the playground, the classroom, and the workplace, culminating in middle age. In this timeline, menopause is the final blow. After women endure decades of messaging that undermines them, here it is yet again, another fundamental female physiological process reduced to evidence for weakness and disease. Viewed through a dark patriarchal lens, in addition to the widely held belief that a woman's age renders her less attractive, the loss of utility in bearing children is an additional unwelcome cultural tax—one that only adds fuel to the fire of inferiority, physically, mentally, personally, and even professionally.

While there is a shortage of reliable science regarding menopause, there is certainly no lack of misleading claims or even misogyny surrounding this topic. In popular culture, menopausal women have often been portrayed through a distressing lens of erratic moods and explosive rages. We're all too familiar with the stereotype of the belligerent menopausal woman, tormented by hot flashes and mood swings, depicted as causing turmoil for her unfortunate and exasperated husband. This view is nothing new. It is deeply rooted in centuries, even millennia, of deep-seated patriarchal mistrust of female bodies. Ready for this?

MENOPAUSE AND THE ANTI-MENOPAUSE MOVEMENT

The first scientific references to menopause originate around the year 350 BC, when Aristotle first observed that women would stop having menstrual discharge sometime between the ages of forty and fifty. However, given that lifespans were shorter back then, not many women had the opportunity to traverse the whole of menopause and live to tell the tale. Besides, in ancient Greece as well as in many other ancient civilizations, a woman's value was linked to her ability to bear children. Those who could no longer do so were evidently not worthy of much interest or study.

Aside from some vague mentions, menopause remained basically invisible to medicine until the nineteenth century. Right around the time male physicians "discovered" women's brains, they also stumbled upon another disconcerting phenomenon: menopause. It might have been overall progress in scientific inquiry, or perhaps that more women were living long enough for menopause to not be ignored, but doctors eventually realized menopause wasn't some kind of freak accident. By then, there were indeed colloquial expressions for menopause all over Europe, such as "women's hell," "green old age," and "death of sex." The word *menopause*, though, entered our vocabularies only in 1821, when French physician Charles de Gardanne came up with the term, borrowing from Greek *men* (month) and *pauein* (to cease or stop), indicating the time at which a woman's period ends.

On brand for those times, the realization that menopause was something worth addressing led clinicians to build a framework for it . . . as an actual disease. A remarkable number of medical conditions, ranging from scurvy to epilepsy and schizophrenia, were readily blamed on this baffling new condition. This should come as no surprise considering the general mindset was that some obscure connection between the uterus and the brain rendered women susceptible to madness, or *hysteria* (from the Greek word *hystera*, meaning uterus). For instance, what we now refer to as premenstrual syndrome (PMS) was thought to be caused by the "suffocation" of the womb filling with blood, or even the upward migration of the womb within a woman's body to suffocate *her*. Clearly, they argued, this unhealthy link will also result in "climacteric insanity" after menopause.

Consequently, drastic and often highly toxic practices emerged to deal with the rebellious wandering womb. Hypnosis, vibrating devices, and blasting the vagina with a jet of water are just a few well-documented techniques. Opium, morphine, and lead-based vaginal injections are others. Then physicians came up with an even more radical solution: surgery. They argued that if the womb was diseased, it should be removed. In hindsight, we now know that *hysterectomies* (the surgical removal of the uterus and ovaries) plunge a woman into menopause almost overnight, potentially worsening its symptoms altogether. So as surgery only exacerbated issues, the asylum beckoned instead. Accounts abound of how women experiencing symptoms of menopause were wrongly diagnosed as "crazy" or "demented," and as such, were locked up in mental institutions. The truth is that these women likely suffered such tragic ends due to the misguided treatments administered by their own doctors.

Fast-forward to the twentieth century. As women gained lifespan, suffrage, and cultural power, menopause finally came to be understood as worthy of medical attention, as opposed to institutionalization. One of the most significant contributions to this shift in perspective came in 1934, when scientists discovered the hormone estrogen. Notably, the term *estrogen* itself was derived from the Greek *oistros*, which means frenzy or mad desire—further reinforcing a historical trend to frame female physiology through the lens of mental instability. Nonetheless, as science moved forward, the link between loss of estrogen and menopause was also found—which led only to updating the definition of menopause to be a disease of "estrogen deficiency." By extension, estrogen became a magical elixir of youth in people's imagination, and as such a profitable drug. Pharmaceutical companies jumped at the opportunity, and estrogen replacement therapy quickly became the treatment of choice for menopause. As recently as 1966, Robert A. Wilson, MD, author of the national bestseller *Feminine Forever*, declared the condition "a natural plague," calling menopausal women "crippled castrates." But, Wilson wrote, with estrogen replacement, a woman's "breasts and genital organs will not shrivel. She will be much more pleasant to live with and will not become dull and unattractive." Later, and perhaps unsurprisingly, evidence emerged that the influential book had been backed by pharmaceutical companies. Not all the propaganda was explicitly sponsored, though—it just spread across culture like wildfire. David Reuben's *Everything You Always Wanted to*

Know About Sex but Were Afraid to Ask (1969) had this to say: "Once the ovaries stop, the very essence of being a woman stops." He added that "a postmenopausal woman comes as close as she can to being a man," correcting, "not really a man, but no longer a functional woman." Little by little, the idea that menopause was an estrogen deficiency syndrome took hold, and it is still common in medical textbooks and practices today.

On the other hand, the actual mechanisms by which estrogen impacts mental health are a strikingly modern discovery. Only in the late 1990s did scientists make a powerful breakthrough: our so-called sex hormones were key not just for reproduction but for *brain function* as well. In other words, the hormones inextricably involved with our fertility, with estrogen leading the charge, turned out to be just as crucial in the overall functioning of our minds. To give you a sense of how recent a finding this is, men had walked on the moon thirty years prior. During those same thirty years on earth, scores of women had been taking hormones in spite of the fact that nobody had a clue about how estrogen really worked from the neck up.

MEDICINE AND BIKINI MEDICINE

Which brings us back to the twenty-first century. Today, menopause is strictly ob-gyn territory, and the connections between our reproductive system and our brain are no longer demonized but are mostly unaddressed. At the same time, in a bizarre turn of events, most scientists now accept that sex hormones are important for brain health, but also believe men's and women's brains to be roughly the same, except for some functionalities involved in reproduction.

Enter one of the major healthcare challenges of our times: bikini medicine. Bikini medicine is the practice of reducing women's health to those body parts found beneath a bikini's confines. It is saying that, from a medical perspective, what makes a woman "a woman" is our reproductive organs and nothing more. Aside from those organs, men and women have been studied, diagnosed, and treated in the same exact way—as if we were all men. This, as it turns out, is not only counter to reality but also destructive in guiding medicine and science to protect women's brains, including those in menopause.

In the simplest terms, the vast majority of medical research has used the male body as its exclusive prototype, "boobs and tubes" notwithstanding. On top of that, as recently as the 1960s, the FDA made it standard practice to deny women of childbearing potential access to experimental drugs and clinical trials, claiming that doing so avoided any potential adverse effects on the fetuses. The phrase *woman of childbearing potential*, however, was taken to mean "any woman capable of becoming pregnant," not solely those who were. This meant that *any* woman from the age of puberty through menopause, regardless of sexual activity, use of contraceptives, sexual orientation, or even any desire to have a child in the first place, was excluded from clinical trials. Where women's brains had been dismissed for centuries as flawed, they were now being rendered invisible for other reasons entirely.

This woman-wide ban was enforced well into the nineties, which means we have decades of medical research based on nearly male-only samples. Shockingly, this is true right up to the present day, as countless drugs have been put on the market that have never actually been tested on women. In fact these drugs often haven't been tested even on female animals. The vast majority of preclinical studies still use only male animals, arguing that variability in sex hormones may "confound empirical findings." This profoundly biased unisex system has been supplying the medical field with data that either doesn't apply or, at best, applies inconsistently to an entire half of the world's population.

Given that the male-dominated medical system has a long history of vilifying menopause while sidelining the study of women's brains, *and* that research has been done mostly on men, *and* that men don't go through menopause, it's really no surprise that the effects of menopause on brain health have remained a mystery—a mystery "solved" with stigma and stereotypes rather than with facts and information. To state the obvious, this has had a catastrophic effect on medical research on the whole, and on the field of women's health in particular.

The consequences are especially clear when it comes to the health of our brains. Because the truth is, women's brains are not the same as men's brains. They are hormonally, energetically, and chemically different. While these differences have no deterministic effects on intelligence or behavior and should never be used to reinforce gender stereotypes, they are crucial to supporting brain health, *especially* after menopause. For some statistics most people aren't familiar with, women are:

- Twice as likely as men to be diagnosed with an anxiety disorder or depression.
- Twice as likely to develop Alzheimer's disease.
- Three times more likely to develop an autoimmune disorder, including those that attack the brain, such as multiple sclerosis.
- Four times more likely to suffer from headaches and migraines.
- More likely to develop brain tumors such as meningiomas.
- More likely to be killed by a stroke.

Notably, the prevalence of these brain conditions changes from broadly equal between men and women *before* menopause to a 2:1 or higher female-to-male ratio *after* menopause. As for the impact of this change, a woman in her fifties is twice as likely to develop anxiety, depression, or even dementia in the course of her lifetime as she is to develop breast cancer. Yet breast cancer is clearly recognized as a women's health issue (as it should be), while *none of the brain conditions above are*. And since breast cancer fits within the "bikini medicine" framework, research and resources have been appropriately devoted to curing it, while hardly any effort has been directed toward menopause care for brain health.

Let's be clear that menopause is not a disease and doesn't *cause* any of the mentioned illnesses. However, the underlying hormonal changes can put a targeted strain on many organs, including the brain, especially when ignored or left unattended. For most women, this can lead to various well-known symptoms such as hot flashes and insomnia. For others, menopause can potentially trigger severe depression, anxiety, or even migraines. For others still, it might be a higher risk of developing dementia down the line. So while the notions of hysteria and womb suffocation were made up, these risks are real. They call for a clear, urgent response: comprehensive research and effective strategies necessary to address the impact of menopause on the brain. Not only do we need help minimizing those initial symptoms, but it's time to accelerate our understanding to prevent the development of more severe issues in the future. Women's medicine must raise its sights—not only beyond the bikini but beyond reproduction as a sole goal. It's time to take an honest and rigorous look at what's happening in women's bodies and brains as a whole, and to fully acknowledge the systemic impact of menopause in the mix.

OUR BODIES, OUR BRAINS

Thus far, we have been looking at the effects of scientific knowledge (and ignorance) at systemic and cultural altitudes. Historically, women have been nothing short of tortured, both physically and psychologically, in the name of menopause. We've been made to believe that menopause can render a woman medically insane, while women of menopausal age and beyond have been rendered invisible in society. This is dangerous, as culture has a powerful effect on how we understand and experience menopause itself—and Western culture has conditioned us to see the symptoms surrounding it as the only meaningful aspects of this transition. While things have certainly improved over time, this trauma has embedded itself into the collective unconscious, influencing not only how a woman is perceived but also how we at times perceive ourselves and our self-worth.

Many women have direct individual experiences with the effects of these frameworks, and not just when going through menopause. Thanks to the one-two punch of bogus beliefs and outdated conventions covered above, our health concerns are routinely downplayed or dismissed. In cardiac care and pain management, for example, it's now a well-documented phenomenon that female patients are much more likely than male patients to be sent home and not treated at all, resulting in poorer outcomes. How does this play out? When they are in pain, women are more likely than men to be told their pain is psychosomatic, hypochondriacal, or stress-related. This sounds like the nineteenth century, but it's happening right now, all too often culminating in a prescription for antidepressants or psychotherapy rather than targeted care.

Given these tendencies, I'm sure you can imagine (or recall) the response to any issues related to menopause being treated as fabricated or unimportant. More broadly, healthcare professionals have often engaged in a disheartening form of medical gaslighting, where they have historically downplayed women's health issues as a whole, and specifically neglected women's concerns around their mental health. As patients, we can therefore grow accustomed to downplaying our own symptoms in turn, for fear of appearing silly or oversensitive or even to avoid being patronized. Unfortunately, brushing off a woman's symptoms can lead to delays in diagnosis and treatment, potentially costing us our quality of life and, if we're unlucky, worse.

As women, we've been taught to fear our hormones and doubt our brains. Women's brain health remains to this day one of the most under-researched, underdiagnosed and undertreated fields of medicine. Not to mentioned underfunded. Women in menopause in particular have been underrepresented and underserved not only in medicine, but also in culture and media. This is seriously overdue for a change—one that I hope science will help bring forth, this time to *support* women instead of harming them.

In this chapter, we address the persistent issue of gender bias in medicine, particularly the exclusion of women, and the inadequate representation of various demographics within the existing research. The glaring neglect of menopausal women in scientific studies is further exacerbated by the insufficient inclusion of women of color, individuals from diverse socioeconomic backgrounds, and those with differing gender identities, among other important factors. This lack of representation is detrimental to us all. Just as it is fundamentally flawed to consider women and men as medically identical, it is erroneous to assume that all women share the same access to well-informed doctors, fitness centers, or nutritious food options. The disparities in access and resources can lead to negative outcomes for brain health, which may in turn affect the experience of menopause. Despite the significance of these considerations, there is a surprising absence of research examining how these factors play out in real-life situations. In an ideal world, accurate information and effortless access to necessary resources and specialists would be available for optimal care throughout our lives. However, given that our world is far from perfect, this book aims to bridge some of these gaps and tackle potential challenges specifically related to menopause. As a scientist, I strive to ensure that my own research addresses these concerns and actively advocate that other investigators adopt a similar approach and interest. By addressing these disparities, we hope to foster a more inclusive and comprehensive understanding of the neuroscience of menopause for all.

In this spirit, I'd like to remind everyone that the field of women's health advances as women's rights evolve. Generations of women have fought for us to have access to healthcare, to be included in clinical trials, to benefit from higher education, and to be acknowledged as lauded contributors in society. Nonetheless, we still strain under the yoke of income, power, representation, and healthcare gaps. It's time to take down the last taboos regarding our bodies *and* our brains and, in doing so, create a culture of understanding, acceptance, and support around menopause. While the work of overcoming the stigma does not fall upon women alone, speaking out loud in our collective voice has the power to yield significant impact. This is a legacy we could be proud to pass onto our daughters and granddaughters, lightening the load for generations to come.

3

The Change Nobody Prepared You For

WHAT IS MENOPAUSE?

After years of discussing menopause with patients, healthcare providers, and the media, I realized there's a great deal of confusion and *misinformation* about menopause. Two things can help bring clarity and reduce worry: (1) clarifying what menopause is and isn't, and (2) separating fact from fiction. Our ideas arrive to us and are transmitted through language. So let's start by looking at terminology, not necessarily as it is commonly used in conversation but rather the way it is used in clinical practice. The most important concepts are summarized in table 1 and described below.

· · ·

Table 1. Glossary: What You Need to Know About Menopause

TERMINOLOGY	MEANING
Premenopause, or reproductive stage	The whole reproductive period before the menopause transition.
Menopause transition	The period before menopause when the timing of the menstrual cycle wobbles and the hormonal and clinical symptoms of menopause begin.
Menopause	The ending of the menstrual cycle. Clinically speaking, the menopause transition is complete after twelve consecutive months since the final menstrual period. There are different ways menopause can occur: it can be spontaneous or induced (see below). All women go through one or the other.
Perimenopause	A phase that starts toward the end of the menopausal transition and continues into the first year after the final menstruation period. You've exited perimenopause and begun menopause once you've had twelve consecutive months without a period.
Postmenopause	The stage starting twelve months after the final menstrual period.
Spontaneous, or "natural" menopause	Menstruation stops when the ovaries run out of egg cells and the production of estrogen and progesterone declines, as part of the aging process. The vast majority of women worldwide will enter menopause aged forty-nine to fifty-two years. Age can differ based on geographical location and ethnic background.
Early or premature menopause	Menopause occurring before age forty (premature) or forty-five (early). It can occur as a result of: ▪ Genetic factors ▪ Polycystic ovary syndrome (PCOS) ▪ Autoimmune disease ▪ Infections ▪ Surgery ▪ Medical treatment
Induced menopause	Menstruation ends due to the surgical removal of the ovaries (*oophorectomy*) or the lapsing of ovarian function due to medical procedures such as chemotherapy or radiation.

(continued)

TERMINOLOGY	MEANING
Surgical menopause	Menopause provoked by surgical procedures. It can occur at any age as a result of: ■ Bilateral oophorectomy: both ovaries are removed. ■ Bilateral salpingo-oophorectomy (BSO): both ovaries and fallopian tubes are removed. ■ Total hysterectomy: the uterus, cervix, ovaries, and fallopian tubes are removed. ■ Note that a partial hysterectomy (removal of the uterus but not the ovaries), ovarian cyst removal, or endometrial ablation does not cause menopause but can affect blood flow to the ovaries, prompting menopausal symptoms at an earlier age.
Medical menopause	Menopause provoked by medical treatments that cause temporary or permanent damage to the ovaries. It can occur at any age, often as a result of: ■ Radiation or chemotherapy ■ Estrogen blockers (tamoxifen): medications that block estrogen's action in specific tissues ■ Aromatase inhibitors: medications that stop estrogen production throughout the body ■ GnRH agonists: medications that keep the ovaries from making estrogen and progesterone, thus stopping ovulation

In medical terms, menopause is the one-year anniversary of your *final menstrual period* (FMP). Long story short, it is confirmed only once you have missed your period for a year or more, which means a yearlong waiting game is required before you can deem your final period genuinely *final*. Then, and only then, are you officially postmenopausal.

While this makes sense from a clinical perspective, this framework can be quite confusing in real life, and for good reason. This description of menopause implies that one will experience a singular moment that starts on a specific day, much like menstruation did some decades prior. You'd think that one day you suddenly stop having your period, and that's that. Many women who have gone through menopause might utter a wry chuckle at this, knowing better. In actuality, menopause is not a day that arrives but a dynamic and sometimes lengthy *process* that can span many years. It is also a time during which whatever your previous sense of normalcy has been, it's now in a state of flux and change.

How Menopause Unfolds: Ages and Stages

The complexity of the menopause transition is just starting to be formalized in medical textbooks, some of which now describe menopause as coming in several phases. In more succinct terms, we are looking at three main stages: premenopause, perimenopause, and postmenopause.

Figure 2. The Three Stages of Menopause

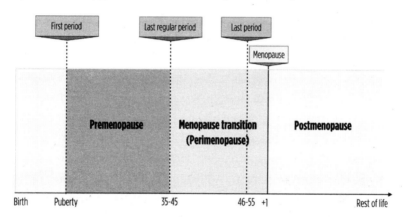

As shown in figure 2:

▶ **PREMENOPAUSE**
As long as you have a regular cycle, you are in the "reproductive" or premenopausal stage. It starts with puberty and ends as the menopause transition begins.

▶ **PERIMENOPAUSE**
Once your period starts becoming irregular, you're entering the menopause transition, which is often called perimenopause. At first, your

period might go a little wonky. It might show up early or late, be longer or shorter, get more or less painful, or be heavier or lighter. In other words, it won't be consistent—everything is up for grabs. And then at some point it won't show up at all for two months or more. At this time, symptoms like hot flashes, as well as possible shifts in sleep quality, mood, and cognition are more likely to flare up, and even the bravest among us may feel they've stayed too long at the fair. The average age that perimenopause starts is forty-seven years, but it varies depending on ethnicity, genetics, and lifestyle factors. The transition usually lasts four to eight years, but can be as long as fourteen years.

▶ **POSTMENOPAUSE**

A full year after your final menstrual period, you are considered post-menopausal. However, let's say you don't have a period for a year, and then, boom, you suddenly have a surprise one—the clock resets, and you are once again in perimenopause! Back at square one, you will again work toward the postmenopausal stage. Importantly, symptoms typically start to recede or disappear a few years after the final menstrual period, though this is not always the case. Most women experience menopause between age forty and fifty-eight, and the average age at menopause is fifty-one to fifty-two. However, the exact timing varies widely from person to person. Additionally, this map applies only to women undergoing *spontaneous* menopause, which occurs when menstruation stops in midlife as a result of the endocrine aging process. Many women experience menopause at younger ages and for different reasons.

▶ **EARLY OR PREMATURE MENOPAUSE**

Some women develop menopause before age forty-five (early menopause) or even before age forty (premature menopause). About 1 to 3 percent of women who experience early or premature menopause do so due to the ovaries producing low levels of reproductive hormones, a condition known as primary ovarian insufficiency (POI). Other women experience menopause prematurely or early because of autoimmune or metabolic disease, infection, or a genetic cause. However, the most common causes of premature or early menopause are surgery and some medical treatments. In this case, menopause is called *induced*, and differs from spontaneous menopause in many ways.

► INDUCED MENOPAUSE

Many women undergo induced menopause, which is when ovulation ends due to either the surgical removal of the ovaries (*oophorectomy*) or the lapsing of ovarian function due to medical procedures such as chemotherapy or radiation. Women who have their ovaries surgically removed while still having a menstrual cycle will find themselves in menopause soon after the intervention. Women whose ovaries stop working for other medical reasons can also develop menopause earlier in life. This is referred to as medical menopause. Surgical menopause may come on very quickly, whereas medical menopause can happen over a time frame of weeks or months. It's important to note that a *partial*, or simple, *hysterectomy*, where the uterus is removed but the ovaries are left in place, will stop menstruation but not ovulation. As such, it will not prompt early menopause. However, hormonal production may decrease, and blood flow to the ovaries may be reduced, too. This may prompt the symptoms of menopause earlier than expected.

How Does Menopause Happen?

To fully appreciate what our bodies experience during menopause, we first need to clarify how hormones function before menopause. During our reproductive years, an intricate dance of hormonal feedback loops occurs approximately every 28 days. The main sex hormones involved are estrogen (the technical term is *estradiol*), progesterone, follicle-stimulating hormone (FSH), and luteinizing hormone (LH). As you can see in figure 3, they rise and drop at varied points during the menstrual cycle, spanning from the first day of your period through the day before your next period.

Figure 3. Sex Hormones During the Menstrual Cycle

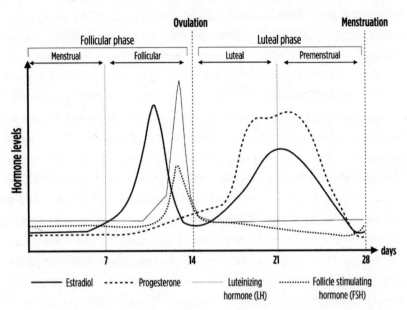

The first half of the menstrual cycle is called the *follicular phase*. At this time, the hormones FSH and LH rise to stimulate the growth of several *follicles*, each containing an egg cell from the ovaries. As the follicles grow, estrogen prompts the growth of the uterine lining to provide the egg with the support it needs to host a baby. Once estrogen levels are sufficiently high, a surge in LH causes the so-called dominant follicle to burst and release the mature egg into the fallopian tube. This process is known as *ovulation*, which occurs mid-cycle. That's when pregnancy is most likely to occur.

The second half of the cycle is called the *luteinizing phase*. If pregnancy has occurred, estrogen and progesterone remain high to prevent the womb's lining from being shed so the placenta can develop. If pregnancy has not occurred, these hormone levels drop instead, prompting the uterus to shed its lining, cuing menstruation.

Although the menstrual cycle is relatively complex, all generally goes to plan as long as these hormones are on the same page, supporting and regulating one another in harmony. That is, until a major event occurs to disrupt this fine-tuned balance: the arrival of menopause.

When a woman is transitioning toward menopause, her ovaries run out of eggs and start producing less estrogen. However, this isn't a linear or steady process, as estrogen doesn't give up so easily.

As you can see in figure 4, estrogen's concentration doesn't drop all at once but can fluctuate wildly as it declines. While not all women exhibit these changes, the "before menopause" part of the graph looks broadly flat. That's because estrogen concentration remains consistent thanks to its levels rising and falling at a regular rhythm with the menstrual cycle. The "after menopause" graph is also virtually flat, as estrogen levels are steadily low at this stage. But the "during" graph looks like the output of a seismograph during an earthquake. As the length and frequency of the menstrual cycle become increasingly irregular during the menopause transition, estrogen's dramatic peaks and valleys make its concentration fluctuate just as widely. Estrogen is not the only hormone that's having ups and downs. As the feedback loops that were so carefully regulating all sex hormones go out of synch, progesterone eventually bottoms out, while FSH and LH increase instead. This hormonal roller coaster can create or contribute to the seemingly random and often unpredictable physical and psychological repercussions many women experience during menopause.

Figure 4. Estrogen Concentration Before, During, and After the Menopause Transition

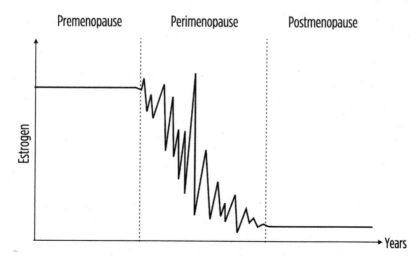

So now we're looking at two ways that the clinical framework for menopause can make the whole process confusing. First off, menopause doesn't happen overnight. Second, while all women experience menopause, every woman's experience is different. Each of us has a unique hormonal fingerprint, a unique reproductive system, and a unique brain. While this individuality has yet to be formalized in medicine, it's clear that both the timeline and the symptoms of menopause can vary greatly from person to person. All of this has led not only to lack of clarity among patients, but also to some widespread inaccuracies around menopause itself, which we'll now proceed to debunk.

MENOPAUSE FAQS

Is menopause an illness or a disease?

Menopause is a physiological stage of life. While the symptoms may not feel normal and the actual challenges surrounding it can feel anything but ordinary, menopause is not an illness, a disease, or a pathological condition. It is a transition. It doesn't need curing or fixing. It does need addressing and managing, if necessary.

Does menopause happen when you're old?

Most women develop menopause in their forties and fifties. On average, menopause occurs around age fifty-one to fifty-two, which is not old by any standards. Besides, recent studies indicate that the actual average age of menopause across the globe is forty-nine, so even earlier. As mentioned already, the exact timing also varies widely from person to person, spanning from the late thirties to the early sixties.

Are blood tests necessary to diagnose menopause?

Since periods become less frequent during the menopause transition and one gets more used to missing them, it may be hard to know when they've stopped for good, leaving many women wondering if they're in menopause or not. I am often asked if there's a simple hormone test that can tell if you're nearing menopause or are already past it. The answer is no. Blood tests can be helpful but are not necessary to diagnose menopause. If you suspect that you're in perimenopause or want to know if you're past menopause, the best thing to do is to have a complete medical examination by a qualified health-care professional. The diagnosis is based on age, medical history, symptoms, and period frequency. Blood work can be used as supportive information, but more often than not, it isn't needed.

Generally speaking, hormone tests are unnecessary to tell if a forty-seven- year-old woman with irregular periods is in perimenopause (most likely she is), or if a fifty-eight-year-old woman with no period for years is postmenopausal (most likely she is). Testing is instead recommended to evaluate fertility problems or when periods stop at an early age, as with POI. Another reason to test is for polycystic ovary syndrome (PCOS), a hormonal condition that can impact menstrual regularity and fertility. Labs may also help determine menopausal status for women who no longer have a period due to medical interventions. These include a partial hysterectomy (the surgical removal of the uterus but not the ovaries) or an endometrial ablation (a procedure that removes the lining of the uterus). These procedures stop your menstrual period but don't stop ovulation. In this case, the occurrence of menopausal symptoms is the first indication of menopause, with blood work providing supporting evidence. In such cases, the levels of estrogen and other hormones, chiefly FSH and another hormone called inhibin B, are measured. Inhibin B regulates FSH production, and it can serve as a marker for ovarian function and follicular content. Normative values are in table 2. When estrogen and inhibin B are low, FSH is high, *and* a woman has not had a menstrual period for a year, it is generally accepted that she has reached menopause. However, a single lab test can be tricky because these hormones may be lower today and higher tomorrow. Their range is quite wide, too. Additionally, a high FSH level in a woman who is having hot flashes and is missing her period does not eliminate the likelihood that she is still in perimenopause. Blood tests are particularly tricky for women in perimenopause, since the hormone levels change throughout the cycle, and the cycle is now irregular, which only increases the variability. In addition, contrary to popular belief, estrogen levels fluctuate widely in perimenopause, sometimes ending up being *higher* than expected rather than lower. Also keep in mind that hormonal contraception such as the pill and some IUDs can stop menstruation and affect the accuracy of the FSH test, making it difficult to determine whether one is past menopause or not.

Table 2. Laboratory Tests for Menopause: Reference Ranges

	PREMENOPAUSE			POSTMENOPAUSE
	Follicular phase	Ovulation	Luteal phase	
Estradiol (pg/ml)	12.4–233	41–398	22.3–341	<138
Progesterone (ng/ml)	0.06–0.89	0.12–12	1.83–23.9	<0.05–0.13
LH (mIU/ml)	2.4–12.6	14–95.6	1–11.4	7.7–58.5
FSH (mIU/ml)	3.5–12.5	4.7–21.5	1.7–7.7	25.8–134.8
Inhibin B (pg/ml)	10–200			<5

Can blood tests predict when you'll go through menopause?

Blood tests cannot predict when you'll go through menopause. When it comes to menopause, there's only one given: at some point, your ovaries will run out of follicles, and you will go through it. Everything else is like that randomly appearing repair person—a bit hard to anticipate. So no, there is no surefire way to predict when you will go through menopause, and certainly not by using blood tests. Rather, your best indicator is . . . your mother. If your mother reached menopause early, late, or somewhere in between, you could eye your calendar with some degree of confidence. The experience and symptoms of menopause are also somewhat similar between mother and daughter, so it is helpful to have this conversation sooner rather than later. Another great indicator of what your menopause will be like, however, is you. The way you experienced puberty and, later on, pregnancy if you have been pregnant, can offer important insights into your menopause journey. We will explore this concept in part 2, but for now consider this: if you experienced mood swings, irritability, or changes in emotional state during puberty, and more so during pregnancy or postpartum, there's a higher chance that you may experience mood disturbances during menopause, too. Similarly, if you experienced hot flashes, sleep difficulties, or brain fog with these reproductive milestones, there is a higher likelihood of encountering them again during the transition to menopause. That said, your experience of menopause is influenced and can be changed by many other factors such as your lifestyle, environment, medical history, and cultural beliefs.

Are blood tests necessary to decide whether hormone replacement therapy (HRT) is indicated?

Blood tests are unnecessary for those aiming to use hormones for symptom relief. This is because we are not treating hormone levels. We are treating the symptoms of menopause, which do not correlate with hormone levels. You may have symptoms even if your hormones are within normal range, and you may have very low estrogen and no symptoms.

Are saliva and urine tests as good as blood tests?

A blood test is the only accurate test for hormonal levels. Saliva and urine tests are often offered to evaluate reproductive hormones but are less precise than blood tests and are not recommended in clinical practice. The well-known DUTCH test (Dried Urine Test for Comprehensive Hormones) is also less reliable than a blood test.

Can HRT be used before menopause?

HRT can be used both before and after menopause. HRT before menopause is typically prescribed to address specific conditions such as POI and other medical indications. Unfortunately, among women without these indications, healthcare providers tend to prescribe HRT only after menopause has occurred, rather than during the perimenopausal phase. From a scientific perspective, HRT was developed to be used in presence of active symptoms, which can be more frequent and disruptive before menopause than after. The decision to use HRT, its timing, and duration should be based on each patient's individual circumstances and needs.

Are there different types of menopause?

There are different types of menopause, chiefly spontaneous and induced menopause, which occur for different causes such as surgery, radiation, or chemotherapy. They are summarized in table 1.

Is it safe to have the ovaries removed?

Oophorectomies are often performed as part of a hysterectomy (when the uterus is removed), the second most common major surgery performed on women in the United States, with only the C-section topping it. Oophorectomy is a first-line treatment for ovarian cancer. Ovarian cancer still kills 14,700 women every year in the United States alone. Removing the ovaries along with the fallopian tubes by means of a procedure called bilateral salpingo-oophorectomy (BSO) is of established clinical benefit when ovarian cancer is found or suspected. It can also be done preventatively in women with a family history of ovarian cancer or proven genetic predisposition, such as specific BRCA gene mutations, and those with medical conditions known as Lynch syndrome and Peutz-Jeghers syndrome. We'll talk more about this in chapter 11.

For now, it's helpful to note that roughly 90 percent of all hysterectomies, which often include the ovaries, are performed for reasons other than cancer. These "benign" conditions include endometriosis, fibroids, benign tumors, cysts, ovarian torsion (the twisting of an ovary), and tubo-ovarian abscess (a pus-filled pocket involving a fallopian tube and an ovary). In such cases, whenever possible, it is common practice to conserve the ovaries during a hysterectomy in women who have normal functioning ovaries. This is because, while oophorectomy is a low-risk procedure, it inevitably results in induced menopause. Therefore, it is a delicate intervention with potential long-term health risks, requiring counseling and a thorough weighing of risks and benefits. In addition, there is accumulating evidence that ovarian cancer may originate in the fallopian tubes, and removing the tubes without the ovaries has been shown to substantially reduce that risk without prompting menopause. Current guidelines for ovarian conservation are summarized in table 3.

There is also some confusion on whether preventative oophorectomies are beneficial to postmenopausal women. While this is a subject of debate, the ovaries continue to make small amounts of estrogen for years after menopause. The ovaries also continue to make two other hormones, testosterone and androstenedione. Muscle and fat cells convert testosterone and androstenedione into more estrogen. Some studies indicate that for women without contraindications, ovarian preservation after menopause might still lower the risk of osteoporosis, heart disease and stroke later in life. As a result, current guidelines recommend ovarian conservation for post-menopausal women with no genetic or additional risks who are undergoing hysterectomy for benign reasons (see table 3).

Despite these revised guidelines, over half of all American women undergoing hysterectomies for these benign reasons still have their ovaries removed along with their uterus. Twenty-three percent of American women aged forty to forty-four and 45 percent of those aged forty-five to forty-nine are still counseled to undergo elective BSO at the time of hyster-ectomy for a benign (noncancerous) condition.

So if you ever find yourself in a situation where you need to have the uterus removed and the surgeon is suggesting that your ovaries be removed, too, but you don't have ovarian can-cer or a genetic predisposition, make sure you discuss the pros and cons of this procedure, considering all aspects of your medical and family history, and clarify why they are rec-ommending it. Keep in mind that there are situations where oophorectomy is indicated even in absence of cancer or cancer risk, and other situations where ovarian conservation is more appropriate.

To be absolutely clear, nobody is telling patients to decline necessary treatment. The point is that oftentimes the possi-ble risks resulting from these surgeries are not made suffi-ciently clear to patients. "I wish I had known" is something I've heard way too many times. It's important to understand what these procedures involve, both in the short and long term, and what treatment options are available, so that each and every woman can make an informed choice for herself and her own health.

Table 3. Bilateral Salpingo-Oophorectomy (BSO): Current Guidelines

Indications for BSO	Suspected or confirmed gynecological malignancy
	Risk reduction surgery (BRCA1 and BRCA2 gene mutations, Lynch syndrome, Peutz-Jeghers syndrome, and a strong family history of ovarian cancer) only after completion of childbearing and over the age of thirty-five
Other indications for BSO	Chronic pelvic pain
	Pelvic inflammatory disease
	Severe endometriosis
Considerations for ovarian preservation	Premenopausal women without genetic predisposition to cancer
	Women with no significant family history of ovarian cancer
	Women with no adnexal pelvic pathology (a lump in tissue near the uterus, usually in the ovary or fallopian tube)
	Postmenopausal women with no additional risk factors

Does menopause affect a woman only physically?

Most certainly not. Menopause is a mind-body experience. When hormones change, we change too. Menopause isn't just a reproductive phenomenon; it impacts a woman's thoughts, feelings, self-image, and behavior. In the next chapter, we'll clarify how many of the symptoms of menopause are in fact a reaction to the brain's own menopausal journey.

4

Menopause Brain Is Not Just Your Imagination

NO TWO MENOPAUSES ARE ALIKE

During menopause, the phase "hot and bothered" takes on a whole new meaning. While generally regarded as a singular event, menopause is more like a syndrome coming with an array of well over thirty different symptoms that appear and disappear according to the woman in question. To make matters even more confusing, one may experience some or none of these symptoms. Generally, a lucky 10 to 15 percent of women report no changes at all aside from irregular menstrual periods that stop when menopause is reached. The vast majority, though, experience several hundred unique symptom combinations.

Further, some symptoms are *somatic*, or of the body, impacting you from the neck down, while others are *neurological*, or from the brain. Notably, the menopause repertoire features at least as many brain symptoms as bodily ones, though it's easy to confuse one with the other. For example, many women think that hot flashes are a sign that there's something wrong with their skin. But the skin has nothing to with that. Hot flashes are triggered by the brain and are a legit neurological symptom. Let's delve deeper into the distinction between these symptom types.

The most common bodily symptoms of menopause are wide ranging and impactful. They include changes in menstruation and period frequency, as well as genitourinary symptoms like vaginal dryness, painful intercourse, stress incontinence, or overactive bladder. Muscular changes manifest as joint pain and stiffness, muscle tension, and aches, while bone-related symptoms include bone frailty and an increased risk of osteoporosis. Breast-related changes can also occur, such as breast soreness, loss of breast fullness, and swelling. However, it's crucial not to overlook the less-discussed bodily symptoms of menopause that can significantly impact women's lives and well-being. These include irregular heartbeat and palpitations, which can be very scary, as well as changes in body composition, weight gain, and slower metabolism, along with digestive issues, bloating, acid reflux, and nausea. Additional changes encompass thinning hair, brittle nails, dry skin, and itchiness; changes in body odor; changes in taste or dry or burning mouth; tinnitus, muffled hearing, or sensitivity to noise; and even the development of new allergies. These symptoms should not be taken lightly, as they can be overwhelming to deal with on their own. Some may even lead to the misconception that your body is betraying you or make you feel as if you're going crazy or losing control.

However, it is the brain-related effects of menopause that typically become the major cause of concern for most women. While some may sound familiar, like the telltale hot flashes mentioned above, others may be surprising (or perhaps you'll be surprised to learn that they also come from the brain). The hormonal chaos of midlife can set off changes not only in body temperature but also in mood, sleep patterns, stress levels, libido, and cognitive performance. Importantly, these shifts can occur without any hot flashes. Furthermore, some women develop neurological occurrences like dizzy spells, fatigue, headaches, and migraines. Meanwhile, others report more extreme symptoms, including severe depression, intense anxiety, panic attacks, and even what's referred to as electric shock sensations. All these symptoms originate not in the ovaries, but in the brain. Yet despite significant progress in understanding the bodily aspects of menopause, we are only just beginning to grasp the full impact of the emotional, behavioral, and cognitive shifts that can arise during this transition. Unfortunately, few women, and perhaps fewer doctors, are fully aware of how common these symptoms are. What many also don't realize is how disruptive, intense, and severe they can be. That's why we are here. In this chapter, we'll go over the core "brain symptoms" of menopause.

It's Getting Hot in Here

While the gradual disappearance of your period might not immediately catch your attention, hot flashes, for one, are hard to ignore. Hot flashes are considered the cardinal feature of menopause, experienced by as many as 85 percent of all women. The medical term for hot flashes is *vasomotor symptoms,* clarifying that they are caused by the constriction or dilation of blood vessels. This results in a sudden rush of heat, usually felt across the face, neck, and chest. Your skin might redden as if you're blushing or mounting a fever, and it's common to break into a sweat just as intensely. If you lose too much body heat at once, you might get chills instead.

Calling this experience a flash, however, is misleading. Here one minute and gone the next? No way. These signs of menopause can last at least a few minutes but can continue for up to an hour, which strains anyone's definition of a flash. Not only do they take their time dissipating once you're having one, but they can stick around in your life for quite some time. The average woman experiences hot flashes for three to five years, but many can have them for ten years or longer. Scientists have identified four patterns when it comes to hot flashes:

- *The lucky few:* About 15 percent of women never have a hot flash.
- *Late-onset hot-flashers:* Women who experience their first hot flash only close to or after their final menstrual period. About a third of all women fall in this group.

- *Early onset hot-flashers:* Women who begin to experience these symptoms several years before their final menstrual period. Fortunately, hot flashes tend to end as the menstrual period does.
- *Super-flashers:* Women who experience hot flashes early in life, with symptoms lasting well past menopause. About one in four women fall into this category. Smokers (past and current) and those who are more than moderately overweight are more likely to be super-flashers.

Ethnicity, lifestyle, and cultural factors likely play a role, too. African American and Afro-diasporic women tend to experience more frequent and severe hot flashes than their Caucasian counterparts, whereas Asian women report fewer, for reasons that are under investigation.

Running the gamut from uncomfortable to unbearable, hot flashes land a one-two punch when they occur at night. In this case, they're colloquially referred to as night sweats. Until they experience them, most people don't appreciate the difference. According to medical textbooks, night sweats are repeated episodes of heavy sweating during sleep, heavy enough to soak your nightclothes or bedding. However, the real-life experience of night sweats is a whole different ball game. According to women experiencing them, night sweats are more aptly described as a five-alarm fire—a throw-off-the-covers, dive-into-an-Arctic-cold-shower kind of experience. These events can be profoundly debilitating, especially as they tend to occur frequently, sometimes more than two or three times a night. This also goes a long way to explaining why menopausal women have a reputation for emotional volatility. When you can't get a decent night's rest for months, let alone years at a time, and you're dealing not only with the flashes but also with clinical-level sleep deprivation . . . being in a bad mood seems unavoidable.

In spite of women's concerning experiences, most doctors persist in thinking that vasomotor symptoms are nothing but a quality-of-life issue. This is not the case. For instance, there is robust evidence that women who experience hot flashes earlier in life might be at higher risk for heart disease. Additionally, night sweats have been linked to presence of white-matter lesions in the brain. These lesions result from a wearing away of the brain's white matter, the connective nerve fibers between neurons. There is some evidence that the more night sweats one experiences, the more white-matter lesions there are in the brain, potentially causing more severe issues down the line. In a nutshell, hot flashes are very real symptoms that need attending to *before* they become an actual problem. At a minimum, reports of severe and frequent vasomotor symptoms should cue doctors to look more closely at a woman's cardiac health, as well as her brain health. Fortunately, there are ways to alleviate, reverse, and even prevent vasomotor symptoms, which we'll review in later chapters.

An Emotional Roller Coaster

Roughly 20 percent of all women experience mood swings and depressive symptoms during perimenopause and in the years immediately after the final menstrual period. While menopause in and of itself does not cause depression, it is pretty efficient at bringing on the blues. Changing hormones can trigger mood swings that make you less able to cope with things you'd normally let roll off your back. Moreover, for some women, these hormonal dips can set off actual depressive episodes, especially for those who've gone through major depression in the past. In such cases, it is possible for symptoms to return during the menopause transition. Additionally, even women who have never encountered depression in their lives may find themselves grappling with it for the first time during perimenopause.

Some of the most common emotional changes associated with menopause include irritability, anxiety, and a diminished ability to deal with life's everyday hassles. Feelings of sadness, fatigue, lack of motivation, and difficulty concentrating can also arise, along with emotional flatness, trouble getting motivated, or a sense of overwhelm. It's not uncommon for crying or other releases to happen more often, more intensely, or seemingly unexpectedly. While less prevalent, some women may even develop panic attacks, while others report feeling downright rage—all easy fodder for the stereotype of the *mad, bad, and dangerous* menopausal woman. Considering what a life with ongoing hot flashes can be like, this moodiness might not be such a mystery. However, menopausal depression often occurs independent of hot flashes or other symptoms.

If you are experiencing mood swings or depressive symptoms, speak with a healthcare provider who can help diagnose whether you are feeling moody, depressed, or stressed out as a result of menopause—or whether you are suffering from clinical depression of other origin. Since menopausal depression and major depression share overlapping symptoms, it's good to get to the bottom of things and receive appropriate care. The good news: Mood fluctuations are treatable. If emotional ups and downs during perimenopause impact your normal daily activities or your relationships, talk to your doctor about options. Thankfully, a variety of treatments are available, including menopause hormone therapy and/or antidepressants, as well as lifestyle adjustments, such as a specifically tailored diet and exercise plan, which we'll discuss in parts 3 and 4 of this book. Also keep in mind that once hormones settle down after menopause, mood fluctuations tend to stabilize, too.

Menopause Can Keep You Awake at Night

Poor sleep quality and sleep disturbances are lesser-known changes during this phase of life, yet they're highly prevalent. While sleep quality naturally declines with age, menopause can add fuel to the fire, turning what would have been a gradual process into a swift kick toward sleep deprivation. By waking you up in the middle of the night, night sweats in particular make for poor sleep if you're lucky and full-blown insomnia if you're not. Then of course, as discussed above, if a person is not sleeping well, mood and mental equilibrium are bound to be affected. Chronic sleep disturbances can trigger not only low mood, anxiety, and potential depression but brain fog and exhaustion, too. Lower estrogen levels further confound your brain, decreasing your capacity to deal with stress in the first place. Even more concerning is that sleep is essential in forming memories, quenching inflammation, and even reducing the risk of cognitive impairment in old age—all of which makes resting our busy minds crucial for the long haul.

It is therefore very important to address sleep disturbances that occur during the menopause transition. Perhaps not surprisingly, perimenopausal and postmenopausal women report more sleep issues than any other segment of the human population. They are also more likely than other people to report spin-off problems such as anxiety, stress, brain fog, and depressive symptoms. According to the Centers for Disease Control and Prevention:

- More than half of all perimenopausal women sleep less than seven hours a night. For context, over 70 percent of premenopausal women sleep more than that—a significant jump.
- One in three perimenopausal women have trouble not only falling asleep but also *staying* asleep, waking up multiple times per night.

For some good news, while several women struggle deeply with sleep throughout perimenopause, many eventually find a new normal, with their sleep improving fairly quickly a few years after they transition to the postmenopausal stage. However, just as many continue to wrestle with poor-quality sleep and oftentimes insomnia. To make matters worse, postmenopausal women are two to three times more likely than premenopausal women to develop new sleep problems, such as sleep apnea. While this disorder is typically considered a men's issue, once menopause kicks off, women are also at increased risk, possibly because of changes in muscle tone. Sleep apnea is a chronic breathing disorder during which one repeatedly stops breathing mid-sleep. Typically, this is due to a partial or complete obstruction (or collapse) of the upper airway, often affecting the base of the tongue and the soft palate, or due to a depressed signal from the brain to initiate a breath. These events can last ten seconds or longer, sometimes occurring hundreds of times per night, causing severe sleep disruptions.

Sleep apnea is more common than you probably think. The National Sleep Foundation reported that it likely affects as much as 20 percent of the population, although as many as 85 percent of individuals with sleep apnea don't know they have it. That seems to be particularly the case for women, for two reasons. First, many women attribute the symptoms and effects of sleep disorders (like daytime fatigue) to stress, overwork, or menopause, rather than to sleep apnea. Second, the symptoms of sleep apnea are often more subtle in women than in men (read, women snore less). As a result, women tend to not seek evaluation for sleep apnea, which in turn delays diagnosis and treatment.

Given the importance of sleep for your health, both physical and mental, I strongly recommend that you get a proper sleep evaluation if you are concerned that your sleep symptoms may be due to menopause, sleep apnea, or a combination of the two. Treatments for sleep apnea are available, which often include lifestyle changes and the use of a breathing assistance device at night, such as a continuous positive airway pressure (CPAP) machine. Sleep disturbances due to menopause are also just as important to address. As with the other symptoms so far, remedies are available, which we'll review in part 4.

Brain Fog Can Spark Fears of Dementia

Along with sweating and poor sleep often comes something many women don't anticipate: brain fog. Few things are more disconcerting than when your brain feels like mush rather than the sharp and useful tool you've been used to, or when your memory takes a turn for the worse. Although *brain fog* is not a medical term, it aptly describes the fogginess in one's thinking, the mental fuzziness, and the difficulty processing information that often accompany menopause. This phenomenon is perhaps best described as feeling that you are enveloped in cotton wool, finding it hard to absorb and recall information or concentrate on everyday tasks, which now require greater concentration, time, and effort. The most common complaints include things like forgetting what you walked into a room for, struggling to remember words and familiar names, or losing focus during a mental task. One of our patients described this experience in these words: "I just don't feel like myself anymore. I feel like a shell of my former self." Another patient told me she was feeling lethargic, almost spent: "No matter what I do, my brain just won't turn on."

According to recent statistics, over 60 percent of all perimenopausal and postmenopausal women struggle with brain fog. The experience is so marked that it can disturb one's sense of efficiency, especially when memory lapses crop up. It's important to realize that forgetfulness can spike during perimenopause, which can feed fears not only of going crazy but of experiencing early dementia. In other words, we are looking at millions of women in the prime of life who suddenly feel like the rug has been pulled out from under them—blindsided by their bodies, let down by their brains, and failed by their doctors, who also may not realize that those are symptoms of menopause.

Here are some examples of what brain fog may feel like:

- Problems with short-term memory; forgetting details like names, dates, and sometimes events; forgetting things that you usually have no trouble remembering (memory lapses); confusing dates and appointments.
- Difficulty concentrating; having a reduced focus or a shorter attention span (easily spacing out).
- Feeling mentally slower than usual (mental fatigue); taking longer to finish things or feeling disorganized, with slower thinking and processing.
- Trouble multitasking, like answering the phone while typing, without losing track of one task; it's harder to do more than one thing at a time.
- Fumbling for the right word or phrase; being unable to find the right words to finish a sentence; losing your train of thought.

- Having trouble following the flow of a conversation.
- Feeling sluggish or tired or lacking energy.

That's the bad news. The good news is that experiencing meno-pausal brain fog or forgetfulness *does not mean* that one is necessarily developing dementia. As a specialist in the field, I want to reassure everyone that there's a big difference between perceiving a decline in brainpower and being clinically impaired. Although the symptoms listed above may inconvenience and challenge you beyond your pa-tience, the power surges and sputters you're experiencing do not mean that the lights are going out (although the "find my phone" app on cell phones may become your new BFF). In all seriousness, in medicine, brain fog is referred to as *mental fatigue*, or more technically, as *subjec-tive cognitive decline*. The key word here is *subjective*. When applied to midlife women, this definition indicates that patients are "aware of a decline from a previous level of cognitive functioning, in the absence of objective impairment." In other words, although you may feel that you're underperforming relative to your usual standards (which in-volve a subjective perception), chances are, your performance is objec-tively within the appropriate reference range—or consistent with that of other people your age.

To give you a better sense of how this plays out, let's say that I asked you to take a test called a Mini-Mental State Exam (MMSE). This test is commonly used to measure cognitive performance. The maximum score is 30. A score of 25 or higher reflects normal cognitive performance. A score of 24 or below indicates possible cognitive impairment instead. The lower the score, the more likely a person is to have dementia.

So let's say that, before "menopausing," you got a score of 30. As you start going through the transition, that 30 may become a 29 or a 28. While that's a small change, one can totally feel it. Appointments may get missed, keys may be misplaced, and names may not come to mind as easily as before. Still, although your performance has indeed de-clined relative to your own baseline, this change does not put you in the "impaired" range, and therefore does not indicate a cognitive defi-cit. For context, consider the brain imaging work we reviewed in chapter 1, showing brain changes before and after menopause. As dramatic as those changes appear, they are not indicative of a brain deficiency. They are a change from a previous level of brain energy. What those scans show is not dementia, but menopause.

So what is really going on? While menopausal brain fog hasn't been the subject of much research, there is robust evidence that typically it is a temporary change, and that mental acuity recuperates after menopause. This phenomenon is well described in one of the most extensive studies thus far, the Study of Women's Health Across the Nation (SWAN). The SWAN traced cognitive performance in over 2,300 midlife women over several years. Many of these women were at the premenopausal stage when the study began. This way, the investigators were able to compare cognitive performance in the same women, before and after menopause, similar to what we do with our brain scans. The results: Over time, as the premenopausal women in the study entered perimenopause, their scores on some cognitive tests did indeed show a decrease. Specifically, the participants had a harder time remembering some information and needed more time to complete some of those tests than before they were perimenopausal. Crucially, the numbers bounced back a few years later, after these same women reached the postmenopausal stage, after which cognitive performance returned more or less to previous scores.

For context, consider the brain imaging work we reviewed in chapter 1, showing brain changes before and after menopause. As dramatic as those changes appear, they are not indicative of a brain "deficiency." They are a change from a previous level of brain energy. What those scans show is not dementia but menopause. As we'll see in the next chapter, our latest studies reveal that in many cases, the perimenopausal declines in brain energy eventually stabilize, too— and that women's brains have the ability to adjust to menopause and carry on.

To sum it all up:

- Women's concerns about their cognitive functions are *legitimate and valid*. If a woman approaching or past menopause feels she is having memory problems, no one should brush it off or attribute it to a jam-packed schedule—or, worse, to "just being a woman."

● Some cognitive slippage is indeed common during the perimenopausal and early postmenopausal years. In most cases, these issues are short-lived and go away over time. While your brain may feel off or muddy for a while, when the transition passes, typically the clouds clear and the fog lifts.

Not to put too fine a point on it, but even during this phase, women *outperform* men on those very same cognitive tests measuring memory, fluency, and some forms of attention. That's true both *before and after* menopause. During the menopause transition, cognitive scores may take a dip, bringing women's performance effectively within men's range. In other words, the average menopausal woman performs just as well as the average man of the same age, who is not, of course, in menopause. (Take that, Darwin!)

With all that said, here's an important caveat. These findings represent an *average* effect. That is to say, the average woman transitioning to menopause may experience some cognitive decline, which may either remain stable or be followed by a rebound. But this word *average* hides the reality that this is not true for all women. In fact, some don't show *any* changes in cognitive performance, which is great. But others show more severe changes, which may be a warning that something serious is afoot. In keeping with the example above, if your MMSE score has gone down from 30 or so to 24 or lower, that is an unusual change that needs further evaluation. Women are not impervious to cognitive impairment— as we discussed, two-thirds of all Alzheimer's patients are women. For some, cognitive performance may indeed deteriorate after menopause and become a diagnosis of dementia later on. Likewise, in our brain imaging studies, some women show less of a change as they go through menopause, while for others, the changes in brain energy as well as in other important functionalities are more severe. This is indeed a red flag for a higher risk of developing dementia later in life. So what all this means for each woman who may worry about brain fog in midlife is that we need to take this information very seriously and take great care of our brains during menopause and beyond.

Alzheimer's disease spurs cloudy thinking, and it, too, manifests with difficulty remembering things, coming up with the right words, and having trouble organizing thoughts. So how are we supposed to tell the difference? Generally, the memory changes that occur during menopause aren't functionally disabling—that is to say, they don't severely interfere with your daily life. They also either remain stable or resolve over time. Unlike the brain fog associated with menopause, Alzheimer's is a progressive disease that worsens over time and interferes with your ability to function and take care of yourself. For context, dementia isn't forgetting where you left your keys. Dementia is forgetting what keys are for.

If your cognitive issues during menopause negatively impact your daily life and don't seem to improve over time or with treatment, whether it be medications or lifestyle modifications, you might want to seek out a neurologist or a neuropsychologist. For instance, if you are three to four years postmenopausal and you are still having serious concerns, this would be a good time to be tested, even if just for peace of mind. I would also recommend joining an Alzheimer's prevention program like ours. Our patients receive thorough medical exams, cognitive testing, and brain scans over time, specifically to evaluate whether there are any risks that need attending to. We then intervene by implementing evidence-based recommendations aimed at supporting cognitive health and reducing the risk of dementia. Many of the therapeutic and lifestyle options we apply in our practice also apply to caring for the menopause brain and are described in this book. As a further resource, our scientific papers are available online, and my book *The XX Brain* is entirely focused on dementia prevention for women.

Not in the Mood

Last but not least, let's talk about sex. In both men and women, desire may decrease with age. However, women are two to three times more likely to be impacted. What causes a lessening of libido can be complex, but it is a common concern with menopause, with as many as 30 percent of women experiencing a drop in desire during those years—an effect that generally peaks during perimenopause and early postmenopause. However, while menopause has long been portrayed as a bummer for sex, recent studies reveal that midlife sexuality is not that tidy after all. While it is true that some menopausal women may gladly give up sex for sleep or chocolate, others report quite the opposite, experiencing renewed interest and desire. This tends to happen during the late postmenopausal phase, typically after age sixty to sixty-five.

While we're still studying the various reasons behind this variability, there are some consistent factors at play. For example, vaginal dryness or atrophy, which is the thinning, drying, and inflammation of the vaginal walls that may occur during menopause, can render sex painful. Other symptoms of menopause, such as hot flashes, insomnia, and fatigue, may also undermine sexual motivation and interest, and sometimes negatively impact self-esteem. In some cases, low libido may be originating in the brain itself, an often-overlooked sign of hormonal turmoil. Let's face it: feeling exhausted, stressed, sleep deprived, and sweaty may not help your appetite for sex.

However, scientists have found that your mindset matters, too. Changes in libido have been linked, at least in part, to a woman's attitude toward sex *before* menopause. If we return to the SWAN project, in another study, investigators worked with 1,390 midlife women for as long as fifteen years, asking them to rate how important sex was to them as they moved through menopause. About 45 percent of women in the survey indicated that sex did indeed become less important to them as they traversed menopause. But the remaining 55 percent either considered sex as consistently highly important or didn't consider sex very important to start with and stuck with that viewpoint throughout their menopause. Interestingly, women who reported having more satisfying sex, both from an emotional and a physical standpoint, were more likely to rate sex as "highly important" at any age. Those more likely to rate sex as "not very important" after menopause also tended to have depressive symptoms, highlighting the impact of emotional health on sexuality, among other things. Additionally, women who underwent surgical menopause showed a more significant decrease in desire, which may be due to their experiencing more abrupt hormonal shifts. There's a lot to consider surrounding this issue; solutions and suggestions will be addressed in upcoming chapters, but as a quick preview, some hormonal and nonhormonal therapies seem to make a real difference, and so does cognitive therapy. If you look at your sexual health as another aspect of your menopause that needs attention, now and for the future, it makes sense to address any sources of disruption. Having a healthy sexual life, if you wish, can be another invigorating aspect of your life during and after menopause.

The Menopause Brain Is Real

Based on all the evidence so far, we are here today to introduce and formalize the concept of *menopause brain*. It is important to redefine and understand it from the perspective of the women who are living through it, rather than through the narrow lens of societal perceptions or outdated clinical practices.

Menopause brain encompasses a range of changes in body temperature regulation, cognition, mood, sleep, energy, and libido experienced during the menopausal transition. It can vary in severity and duration among individuals, and not all women will experience these changes. The most common symptoms that collectively contribute to menopause brain include:

- Hot flashes: Sudden feelings of intense heat accompanied by sweating, rapid heartbeat, and flushing of the face and upper body.
- Sleep difficulties: Disrupted sleep patterns, insomnia, or fragmented sleep.

- Mood changes: Mood swings, irritability, anxiety, or feelings of sadness or depression.
- Memory lapses: Memory issues, such as forgetfulness or having trouble recalling names, dates, or details.
- Difficulty concentrating: Reduced focus and attention span, increased distractibility.
- Slower cognitive processing: Mental fogginess or sluggishness, trouble thinking clearly, more difficulty processing information or making decisions.
- Word retrieval problems: Trouble finding the right words or expressing thoughts verbally.
- Decreased multitasking abilities: Difficulty juggling multiple tasks or switching between tasks, leading to feelings of being overwhelmed.
- Low energy: Fatigue, lack of motivation, and decreased overall energy levels.
- Low libido: Decreased sexual desire or interest in sexual activity.

We've established that the menopause brain is anything but a breeze. The symptoms that may crop up during this life stage are very real and need addressing. However, we don't just have problems; we have solutions! No woman needs to suffer unnecessarily because of menopause. For one, we can feel a welcome relief discovering that several symptoms that appear during the transition can just as often spontaneously disappear after menopause. Having the variety of our experiences and concerns validated also holds power and comfort in and of itself. The postmenopausal stage of a woman's life is not the "over and out" that society has mistakenly signaled. Instead, it can come with relief and renewed energy, not to mention a broader outlook on life.

Armed with this reassurance, we will now clarify how and why menopause impacts the brain and the significance of this impact for women's health. This information is key for understanding menopause and for choosing the best way to manage this important transition. In fact, the symptoms of menopause can not only be reduced but often entirely eliminated by following the program outlined in the chapters to come. It is easier to then find further comfort in the prescription treatments available to us, along with appropriate natural remedies and lifestyle modifications. Postmenopausal women will also greatly benefit from these guidelines, which are proven to protect and invigorate the mind at any age.

PART 2

THE BRAIN-HORMONE CONNECTION

5

Brain and Ovaries: Partners in Time

THE BRAIN-OVARIES CONNECTION

The human brain may well be the most complex biological structure on Earth. With its estimated 100 billion neurons and 100 trillion connections, it's the crown jewel of our species and the source of all the qualities that make us human. It is the seat of intelligence, the interpreter of the senses, the supervisor of behavior, and the initiator of body movement.

To achieve all this, the brain is in close contact and integrated with every other part of the body, and very much shaped by all these interactions in return. For women, one of the most extraordinary and consequential connections is between our brain and our ovaries, its depth becoming clear when we take a peek at evolution. The survival of a species ultimately depends on reproduction and the relaying of its genes to future generations. Our body is optimized to support this capability, with the brain in the driver's seat. This is important because human reproduction is complex, involving the many physiological, emotional, and behavioral interactions necessary to select a reproductive partner and then maintain the relationships that make it easier to raise offspring. As a result, the female brain has evolved to be not only intricately wired for reproduction but also deeply integrated with our ovaries to ensure all these mechanisms are in place.

THE NEUROENDOCRINE SYSTEM
AND ITS ROUTES

These crucial connections are powered by the *neuroendocrine system,* a network that connects the brain to the ovaries and to the rest of our hormonal system, the complexity of which reveals a level of teamwork between these organs that few have sufficiently fathomed. That's where we come in. Thanks to the close monitoring of estrogen by these regions, the brain can coordinate the myriad physical and mental functions necessary for reproduction and beyond. Straight ahead, a little primer: Neuroendocrine System Anatomy 101.

Route 1. The HPG
(Hypothalamic-Pituitary-Gonadal Axis)

Envision this system as a subway map with several stations, the brain at one end and the ovaries at the other, as we spotlight the most important routes and stops. The ovaries (aka gonads) are so strongly wired to the brain, specifically to two structures called the pituitary and hypothalamus, that medical textbooks identify these connections as a single entity: the *hypothalamic-pituitary-gonadal axis,* or HPG. The HPG is the pillar of the neuroendocrine system, dedicating itself to regulating reproductive behavior at all stages of life. As shown in figure 5, eight major glands are part of the HPG. Picture each gland as a stop on Route 1.

1. Pituitary gland. The first station on the HPG is the *pituitary gland.* The size of a pea, this small but mighty gland has a big job: it makes hormones that regulate the activity of all the other glands, the ovaries included. As a matter of fact, the most important hormones produced by the pituitary are FSH and LH—those same hormones that prompt ovulation during our reproductive years. The pituitary is also involved in making *oxytocin* (responsible for contractions during labor and lactation afterward), *vasopressin* (in charge of blood and water volume), and *growth hormones* (promoting the development of the entire human body, brain included).

2. Hypothalamus. This gland monitors the entire nervous system on behalf of the pituitary gland and flags anything requiring its special

Figure 5. The Neuroendocrine System

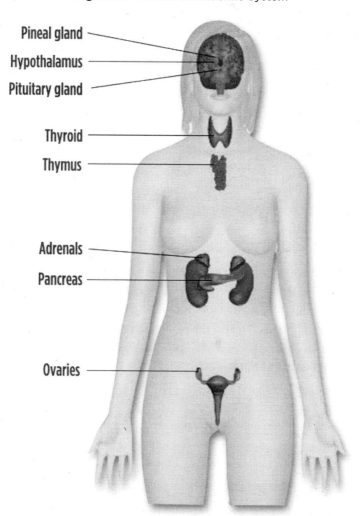

attention. This gland is a big deal, as it's in charge of stimulating the production of LH and FSH by the pituitary, which results in the production of estrogen and progesterone in the ovaries. You could say it's also head of homeostasis, controlling body temperature, sleep patterns, appetite, and blood pressure, therefore maintaining the body's overall balance.

3. Pineal gland. Located in the brain's very center, this gland receives and conveys information about our environment's current light-dark cycle and secretes the hormone *melatonin* accordingly. Like Mr. Sandman, we count on it to signal sleep.

4. Thyroid gland. Down in the neck, this butterfly-shaped beauty regulates metabolism and temperature. The thyroid produces two hormones you're likely familiar with from your blood-test results: T3 (triiodothyronine) and T4 (thyroxine). Attached to the thyroid are four glands no larger than a grain of rice, called the *parathyroids*. These tiny glands attend to calcium regulation, which is important for bone health.

5. Thymus. Located in the upper chest, the thymus is like a bodyguard, producing white blood cells to fight infections and give abnormal cells the boot.

6. Pancreas. This organ-gland complex acts as a liaison between the hormonal and the digestive systems. The pancreas produces enzymes to assist digestion while also making two essential hormones to control the amount of sugar in the bloodstream, like the famous *insulin*.

7. Adrenal glands. This dynamic duo sits on top of your kidneys, producing hormones involved in regulating your metabolism, immune system, blood pressure, and stress response. Their claim to fame is adrenaline, a hormone that stops the body from caving during moments of flight or fight, but can also give you a burnout.

8. Ovaries. We reach our final station—the ovaries. In addition to holding the egg cells necessary for reproduction, the ovaries produce estrogen and progesterone under the hypothalamus's supervision, as well as testosterone.

By examining the HPG pathways and its crucial components, we can see how this intricate system not only prepares the entire body to potentially host a pregnancy but also supports a range of behaviors leading up to that significant moment, from the sensation of butterflies in your stomach to feeling energized during a romantic courtship. In addition, by acting upon this system, estrogen in particular has been shown to boost metabolism, protecting us against weight gain, insulin resistance, and type 2 diabetes. Estrogen is also instrumental in maintaining bone health and in supporting the heart by keeping blood vessels healthy, possibly by keeping tabs on inflammation and cholesterol levels. On the downside, this connection is also responsible for the many physical, or bodily, symptoms experienced with the arrival of menopause. For instance, the risk of diabetes, osteoporosis, and heart disease all increase after menopause. Yet for all the good that estrogen does for a woman's body, that's nothing compared to what it does for her brain. So on to the next, and much less appreciated, brain-hormone route: inside the brain itself.

Route 2. The Brain-Estrogen Network

The neuroendocrine system doesn't stop with the HPG. As shown in figure 6, it communicates with many other key regions of the brain,

Figure 6. The Brain-Estrogen Network

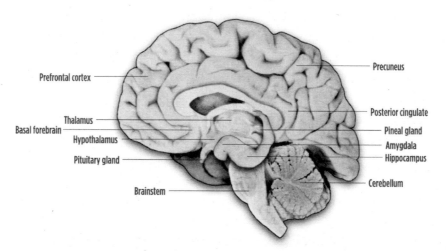

which are referred to as the *brain-estrogen network,* as they are also susceptible to estrogen levels. The most notable stops on Route 2 are:

1. Limbic system and brainstem. The limbic system is buried deep within the brain, snuggled just above the brainstem, which connects our brains to the spinal cord running down the rest of the body. Traced back to our evolutionary roots, these ancient parts of the brain are trained on instinctive behaviors and emotional responses. These impulses include stress, appetite, sleep/wake, feelings, and nurturing instincts.

2. Hippocampus. This seahorse-shaped structure is considered the memory center of the brain. Located in the limbic system, it is responsible for forming episodic memories, or memories of things you did in the past, like experiences from your childhood or your first day at work. The hippocampus also creates associations between our memories and our senses, connecting summer with the smell of roses—while helping us learn new things and aiding our sense of direction.

3. Amygdala. The hippocampus's BFF, the amygdala, plays a central role in emotional responses, including feelings like pleasure, fear, anxiety, and anger. The amygdala also strengthens our memories with emotional content.

4. Cingulate cortex and precuneus. These neighboring regions of the brain's cortical mantle are important for emotional processing, learning, social cognition, and autobiographical memory. The latter refers to our capacity to recall our personal history and events, like what we did on a specific date at a specific time.

5. Prefrontal cortex. This is a super-evolved section of the brain that helps us set and achieve goals. The prefrontal cortex assesses information from multiple brain regions and adjusts behavior accordingly. Doing so contributes to a wide variety of executive functions, including focusing one's attention, controlling impulses, coordinating emotional reactions, and planning for the future. A heavy hitter, the prefrontal cortex is also involved in memory and language.

To summarize, the highly specialized HPG and brain-estrogen networks ensure that our brains and ovaries are closely connected, on an hour-to-hour basis, and that this connection has wide-ranging effects not only on the body but also on our emotions, sensations, and ability to think and remember. As a result, *the health of the ovaries is linked to the health of the brain, and the health of the brain is linked to the health of the ovaries.* Western medicine separated a woman's brain and ovaries into different disciplines and practices, but no woman in the world has the luxury of separating them in her own body. The hormones flowing back and forth between them spur these organs to develop as partners: they mature together, cross milestones together, and in many ways, age together, too. Thanks to just how far-reaching this interconnectedness is, any changes in hormonal quantity and quality can profoundly affect not only a woman's reproductive health but also her physical and mental health.

THE FEMALE BRAIN RUNS ON ESTROGEN

Throughout the book, I am trying to reinforce the idea that there's much more to estrogen than fertility. Beyond its role in reproduction, this versatile hormone is involved in a number of brain processes. That's because the brains of people born with ovaries, scientists have learned in recent decades, are genetically engineered to respond preferentially to the estrogen made by said ovaries.

As it turns out, day in and day out, estrogen molecules slide right into the brain, searching for special receptors that are shaped precisely for this hormone. The receptors are like tiny locks, waiting for the right molecular key (estrogen) to turn them on. This is a vivid image for a crucial idea: women's brains are hardwired to receive estrogen. Once it arrives, estrogen latches on to these receptors, activating a windfall of cellular activities in the process. Loaded with these receptors, our brains are ready-made to be estrogen-fueled.

A knowledge of this and of the workings of the neuroendocrine system makes it easier to understand how menopause can set off such a wild cascade of brain effects. If you're a typical woman moving through your forties or fifties, your lifetime egg supply is running out; as that happens, the intricate, multi-hormone reproductive-signaling loop grows confounded, its triggers altered by the biology of change. Meanwhile, as the brain and ovaries start misreading each other's demands for action, the brain frantically cranks up estrogen production or accidentally drops the ball instead, effectively throwing the brain-ovaries loop . . . for a loop. Eventually the ovaries stop making estrogen, and what used to be a long-term relationship comes to an end. The symptoms of menopause are then the challenging consequences of a brain full of receptors, receiving less and less of the fuel they need to take action.

It's worth mentioning here that while women's brains are wired to respond to estrogen's activation, men's brains are similarly calibrated for testosterone. This is important, as the quantity and longevity of each sex's activator hormone differ, and testosterone doesn't generally run out until late in life. This more gradual tapering-off process leads to andropause, the male equivalent of menopause. However, as the tabloids remind us, most men remain fertile until their seventies—which in a nutshell means that the testosterone receptors in men's brains have more time to adjust. Women's brains, on the other hand, don't have that luxury.

As science has come to learn, the interaction between estrogen and women's brains is quite complex and easily disrupted. For starters, estrogen itself isn't as simple as it seems. The term "estrogen" actually refers to estrogens—not a single hormone but a class of hormones with similar functions. In chapter 3, I mentioned that the type of estrogen we measure in blood is called estradiol. Estradiol is one of the main three types of estrogen. The other two are called *estrone* and *estriol*.

- Estradiol is the most potent and abundant type of estrogen during a woman's reproductive years and the principal growth hormone required for reproductive development. It is produced mainly by the ovaries, and its levels are markedly reduced after menopause.

- Estrone is made by fat-rich adipose tissue and has a weaker effect than estradiol. After menopause, estrone is the main type of estrogen women's bodies continue to produce.
- Estriol is the estrogen of pregnancy. It is present in nearly undetectable amounts whenever one is not pregnant.

When doctors talk about estrogen, they are usually referring to the combined effects of all three types. But when we're talking about the interaction of estrogen with our brains, we are talking mainly about estradiol.

Estradiol: The Master Regulator of the Female Brain

Estradiol is so instrumental in a seemingly endless list of brain processes that it has gained the title of master regulator of the female brain. I can't help but view estradiol as CEO of the Female Brain, Inc. It's a genius commander in chief who knows all aspects of the business, inside and out. Estradiol's most important functions include:

- *Neuroprotection.* Estradiol plays a defensive role on our behalf by boosting the immune system and imbuing brain cells with the ability to overcome damage and aging.
- *Cell growth.* Not only does estradiol protect the brain cells we already have, but it helps grow new ones, while simultaneously prompting cell repair and new connections throughout the brain.
- *Brain plasticity.* Estradiol boosts the brain's ability to respond and adapt to all sorts of changes, from updating our neuronal networks for learning and memory to preserving the brain's ability to function in the face of damage.
- *Communication.* This hormone has its hands in many pies, impacting multiple *neurotransmitters*, the brain's chemical

messengers for signaling, communicating, and processing information.

- *Mood.* Estradiol has a positive effect on *serotonin*, a mood-balancing chemical that promotes happiness and pleasure, not to mention sleep. It also happens to be "nature's Prozac," delivering an antidepressant effect system-wide.
- *Protection.* Estradiol supports the immune system and protects the brain from *oxidative stress* caused by harmful free radicals that can foster illnesses like inflammatory disease, cancer, and dementia.
- *Cardiovascular health.* Estradiol has positive effects on blood pressure and circulation, protecting both brain and heart against vascular damage.
- *Energy.* This hormone also ensures that glucose, the brain's main meal, is efficiently burnt as energy. Consequently, when estradiol is high, brain energy follows. By charging up brain function, estradiol influences everything from mobility to our cognitive abilities.

So far, so good. However, after menopause, estradiol leaves. She announces her retirement, firmly sets a course to wind down, and kicks up her heels. Estrone is then promoted to the task. Unfortunately, estrone can't do what estradiol did. Without estradiol in town, the brain is driven to distraction. The connections between neurons aren't powered as efficiently as before and tend to slow down. Over time, more connections are lost than renewed. Brain cells experience more wear and tear with less access to repair, which makes them age faster, too. Those happy and calming chemicals that kept our systems balanced don't show up as often as before. It's also more difficult to keep free radicals at bay, rendering the brain more vulnerable to inflammation, aging, and a variety of medical conditions. Bottom line, the loss of estradiol can be so impactful as to, at least temporarily, scramble the mind's once-successful choreography of thought, emotion, and memory.

THE UPS AND DOWNS OF MENOPAUSE

The effects of estradiol's mercurial behavior are particularly felt in the brain regions powered by this hormone, which experience these effects firsthand. The hypothalamus is the central node of this connection and takes the brunt of the impact. Since this gland controls body temperature, an instability in the supply of estradiol means that the brain can't regulate body temperature correctly. Remember the hot flashes? Scientists believe that's the hypothalamus going bonkers.

On top of losing hold over our internal temperature, the brain falters in the regulation of sleep and wakefulness. The result: we have trouble sleeping, with changes in our sleep rhythm and patterns. And since all these brain regions are in communication, the issues between the two can combine and whip up night sweats. The emotional amygdala or its neighbor, the memory-minding hippocampus, take their turns, too—prompting mood swings, forgetfulness, or both. The same goes with the prefrontal cortex, in charge of thinking and reasoning. Maybe the fog rolls in, and you have difficulty focusing or paying attention, or perhaps words don't come to mind as easily as they used to. And let's not forget the perpetual search for that elusive phone!

When we pull back the curtain on what's going on inside the menopaused-out brain, some of its more peculiar symptoms suddenly don't seem so strange anymore. The brain changes we reviewed at the beginning of this book likely make more sense, too. They are a reflection of the brain's attempts to deal with the massive hormonal upheaval and accompanying remodeling underfoot. They suggest that as the brain is busy trying to cope with the consequences of the loss of estradiol, its defense mechanisms are temporarily lowered. The powerful shifts in brain chemistry and metabolism may then prompt the symptoms of menopause, while also rendering some women's brains more vulnerable to a variety of medical stresses such as depression and cognitive decline.

With all that said, there's more to menopause than its downsides. In fact, we've finished reviewing what could go *wrong* with menopause. It's time to explore what could go *right*.

First off, menopause is a window not only of vulnerability but also of *opportunity*, as it provides a critical time to detect any signs of medical risk and to intercede with strategies to reduce or altogether prevent that risk. By knowing *when* to look (during menopause) and *what* to look for (the brain changes and symptoms that can ensue), we can not only validate women's experience of menopause but also address what to do about it. Taking better care of our brains during these years will serve both to bring the symptoms of menopause under control and to dramatically reduce any potential risk of future issues.

Just as important, while many women are vulnerable to neurological shifts during menopause, the majority of the female population gets through this transition without developing severe long-term problems. As we discussed in the previous chapter, symptoms like brain fog and hot flashes tend to ease and eventually fade away a few years into menopause. Personally, these considerations changed my approach to menopause and the focus of my research. Like most other scientists, when I started researching menopause, my initial goals were to understand the symptoms and health risks that menopause can bring about. I was looking for all sorts of things that could go wrong—energy declines, the loss of gray matter, Alzheimer's plaques . . . all the baddies for which we wanted to find solutions. After all, entire bodies of literature portray menopause as a medical mess. But if menopause was such a catastrophe, no woman would be able to remain functional for another thirty years and beyond. So, my team and I set out to investigate.

We enrolled more participants and did even more brain scans. We gathered our data and sifted through it, determined to take in the bigger picture. Over time, as we dug deeper and broadened our sights, we learned about *the good* of menopause—not just the bad and the ugly that's been the takeaway thus far. What we discovered is a broader and bolder story, one that in many ways turns out to be encouraging. I will share more about this in the next chapters, but for now, I want to show you some of our recent work providing evidence that menopause isn't all about vulnerability.

If you recall from chapter 1, our first discovery was that brain energy declines during the menopause transition. I am happy to report that we've made significant progress since those first before-and-after scans were taken. By expanding our studies both in size and duration, we found that, in some brain regions at least, the energy changes appeared to be *temporary*. For instance, while brain energy showed a dip during perimenopause and early postmenopause, its levels stabilized or improved years later. As shown in the figure below, some parts of the brain even showed a refreshing rebound in energy during the late postmenopausal stage, which starts approximately four years after the final menstrual period. Check out the arrows pointing to the frontal cortex below. Remember, this is the brain's thinking and multitasking area.

Figure 7. Brain Energy Changes from Premenopause to Late Postmenopause

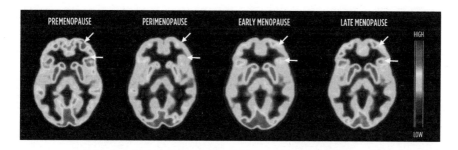

The menopause story brightened further with a late but lovely postmenopausal recoup in the brain's gray matter. While gray matter tends to decline from the premenopausal to the postmenopausal stage, in some brain regions, this change appeared to plateau for quite a few women once menopause was completed. This also correlated with better memory after menopause. Do you remember how memory can decline during perimenopause, returning to close-to-baseline levels later on? Our data are right in synch with this timeline.

It's important to underline that these are recent findings, all in the process of being confirmed on a global scale to reach firm and exact conclusions. While we work to make this happen, my takeaway is that menopause is a dynamic neurological transition that reshapes the landscape of the female brain in unique ways. There are hints and glimmers that this reshaping may include adaptations that help compensate for and maintain brain function, despite the drop in estrogen. In other words, the ovaries may close up shop, but the brain has its ways of carrying on. Many lines of evidence indicate that women's brains have the remarkable, much underestimated, yet-to-be-celebrated ability to *adapt* to menopause. This information is just the beginning of unlocking menopause's secrets and upgrading our experience of this important milestone in every woman's life.

6

Putting Menopause in Context: The Three P's

PUBERTY, PREGNANCY, AND PERIMENOPAUSE

As women, we are used to dealing with hormonal changes. Whether it is puberty, your monthly cycle, the postpartum period, perimenopause, or postmenopause, we experience the ups and downs of hormones for most of our lives. So now that we've reviewed the neuroendocrine system and its star hormones, let's talk about the peak life transitions that distinguish that system and their interconnectedness. Many women go through a trio of these stages in their lives. I like to refer to them as the Three P's: puberty, pregnancy, and perimenopause. These turning points represent moments when our brains and hormones meet and morph in a uniquely female way. While we're all familiar with the idea that our bodies change with these transitions, it's not as obvious how much our brains have to do with them, too. Here's a preview.

Estrogen levels balloon during puberty, plateau as we enter adulthood, and fluctuate with every menstrual cycle, only to peak once again if one gets pregnant. More precisely, hormonal fireworks occur *every time* a woman is pregnant, dipping dramatically once the baby is born. Hormone levels rise again afterward, steering a more or less steady course until reaching the most turbulent of the big P's: peri-menopause. Eventually perimenopause passes, too, and estrogen re-cedes, while other hormones increase instead. We often visualize this hormonal activity as ovary-driven, but our brains would beg to differ. Throughout all these years, our brains are buckled in beside our ova-ries on a serious hormonal roller coaster, making for a just as serious mind-body ride.

In fact, the Three P's are like three peas in a pod; they are part of a continuum and have a lot in common. Looking at their commonalities is particularly helpful to put menopause in context. When we do, we see menopause isn't as alien an event as we've been conditioned to believe but rather another stage of a woman's reproductive *and neuro-logical* journey. Moreover, when we view each of these stages the way brain scientists do, we notice that they each represent a time of vulner-ability (manifesting as symptoms and medical risks) and resilience (including symptom recovery and personal growth). As we explore the latest science on the Three P's, let us remember this age-old adage: Every rose has its thorn.

THE BRAIN FROM BIRTH THROUGH PUBERTY

Most people think a newborn's brain is like a blank slate, ready for the world to write upon it. According to a large body of scientific evidence, however, that's not entirely the case. Brain development, prompted by our DNA, starts in utero, kicking off before we're born. Fun fact: At first, all children's brains appear exactly the same—female. Yes, you heard right. *Female* is nature's default brain setting. (Take that, too, Darwin.) It's only after a surge in testosterone that boys' brains begin to take on male attributes, which, if you recall from the previous chapter, means they become wired to respond more to testosterone.

Over time, estrogen and testosterone play an essential role in the sexual differentiation of the brain, as the structures belonging to the neuroendocrine system begin to differ somewhat between the sexes in their anatomical structure, their chemical makeup, and even in their reactions to stressful situations. While these differences do not dictate sexual preferences or behavior, they are important, as they influence the way our brains mature and eventually age.

At birth, a child's brain contains 80 to 100 billion nerve cells, while new connections between neurons develop at the explosive rate of up to 2 million per second, prompting the brain to quickly almost double in volume. After this impressive upsurge, brain density has reached its max and begins to decrease. A process of refinement and reduction sets in as the brain starts to respond to life experiences and the world around us. Pruning is the process by which a deep restructuring occurs as the most used connections between cells strengthen and take hold and those that are less essential die off. In a perfect example of "use it or lose it," many of the brain's original neurons are discarded, while many more multiply and grow as the child starts engaging with the environment. Keep this process in mind—it is very important to understand menopause as well.

By age six or seven, this elaborate dance of growth and elimination becomes evident outwardly as the child masters new cognitive capacities like reading, tying their shoes by themselves, socializing, and much more. At this point, the brain has reached approximately 90 percent of its full size, and with it, a certain stability in behavior. However, even though it may not grow much size-wise afterward, it is far from done maturing. In fact, most brain regions are still in a state of growth and change, a process that peaks just in time for the first P on our list—the pimple-faced period of emotions run wild: Puberty with a capital P!

HOW PUBERTY CHANGES THE BRAIN

When we hit puberty, the doors fly open at hormone central. During this time, boys' bodies produce significantly more testosterone than girls', while girls' bodies shift into a higher estrogen-to-testosterone ratio. These hormonal surges provoke the body to develop into its adult form, complete with a mature reproductive system. But more is going on than this. This very same hormonal turmoil is also priming the brain for both growth and new forms of learning.

What may come as a surprise is that instead of the brain continuing to grow in size as it matures, it literally *shrinks* during puberty. The neuron-pruning process goes into overdrive once sexual maturation is reached: about half of the brain's original neurons are shed, and their connections are dramatically scaled back. While this downsizing can appear counterintuitive at first glance, it is not only normal but necessary. It's all about the brain becoming leaner and meaner, and more efficient overall. Keeping neurons alive and functioning requires a tremendous amount of energy, so ideally, the brain strives to achieve its goals with as few neurons as possible, working smarter, not harder. This is also how the brain begins to automate specific actions. For example, a teenager can tie her shoes and ride a bike automatically. The neurons initially responsible for breaking down and directing these skills in steps appropriate for a toddler are no longer necessary and can be discarded. The phrase "It's just like riding a bike" is apropos here. Hence, this system consolidation clears out the old and makes room for the new in one fell swoop.

This process is, however, not particularly straightforward, with changes developing at varying rates across different parts of the brain. There's an important back-to-front mismatch in brain development: the amygdala and hippocampus, which are in charge of emotion and memory, kick into high gear early on. The prefrontal cortex—the area in charge of controlling impulses and executive skills, like being self-possessed enough to say, "I'd better not do that"—is late to the party. Since adolescents are working with a frontal cortex still under construction, their self-control is not as accessible as their parents might wish, giving us a peek under the hood regarding the tumultuous moments of recklessness and moodiness of the teenage years. Never fear; this, too, shall pass. As the prefrontal cortex further develops, teens become better equipped to resist impulses and assess potential risks. At the same time, they develop the ability to put themselves in another person's shoes, a capacity that is often called *theory of mind*, or mentalizing. This uniquely human superpower allows us to understand other people's intentions and beliefs. In doing so, we can extrapolate from this data to understand and predict behavior while also better integrating ourselves into society. Today, scientists attribute this remarkable capacity to the puberty-fueled brain revamp. (Hint: This perspective also provides us with a preview of what lies ahead with the next two P's.)

Interestingly, the brain maturation timeline is somewhat different for boys and girls, hitting peak production when children approach sexual maturity, which is around age eleven for girls and fourteen for boys. Perhaps as a result, adolescent girls tend to exhibit earlier and stronger connections between the impulsive amygdala and the cautious-minded frontal cortex than their male counterparts. Whether due to nature, nurture, or both, these differences have been interpreted as evidence that girls mature faster than boys, showing a slight advantage in theory of mind tasks, empathy, social competence skills, and social understanding. They also show better communication abilities, learning to speak at an earlier age and generally reaching a greater fluency—a difference that can persist throughout the lifespan. Lest we fall into stereotyping, let's be clear: We don't review this data to fuel a competition but to better understand women's natural strengths and comprehend how these abilities might develop early in life and then be impacted by aging and reproductive changes. Because sure enough, although exciting new skill sets are being forged, there is a price to pay.

The "Period Brain"

Puberty marks the onset of the menstrual cycle, which can profoundly alter the circuitry of a teen girl's brain, impacting the way she thinks, feels, and acts on a monthly basis. The notion that a woman's cycle can befuddle her brain is a main staple of popular culture. Dismissive and often derogatory statements like "She must be PMS-ing" are by now part of the everyday vernacular. As unsympathetic as these expressions can be, many women do experience a vulnerable side during their period. But while that's made it into society's wry water-cooler rhetoric, the flip side has not. The "period brain" is not all bad news.

Thanks to an incredibly complex neurological phenomenon, the brain's size, activity, and connectivity shift monthly, if not weekly, in synch with our cycle. While these brain micro-cycles are generally subtle, they are quite real. For example, when estradiol runs higher during the first half of the month, brain cells visibly sprout new spines that reach out and connect with other cells, striking up sharpened neuronal conversations near and far. The amygdala and hippocampus swell appreciably in size, and their connections with the prefrontal cortex appear to get stronger—which has been linked to better executive skills and helps us feel more focused and overall more on. Certain cognitive skills are also heightened at this time, such as verbal fluency, communication, and social responsiveness.

On the flip side, as estradiol recedes during the second part of the cycle, some connections between neurons also recede. This has been linked to low mood, irritability, headaches, and even fatigue or sleepiness for some women, while others can feel sad or tearful. These monthly back-and-forths are important to consider because they clarify the very nature of the brain-hormone connection during our reproductive life, while also giving us a preview of what our nonreproductive life might be like, once the menstrual cycle has ended for good. Additionally, the surging hormones of puberty and their fluctuations during a girl's monthly period can render her brain more vulnerable to stress, anxiety, and moodiness. It's telling that the prevalence of depression, anxiety, and eating disorders shifts from being equal between girls and boys before puberty to a 2:1 female-to-male ratio afterward. Moreover, one out of four women suffers from clinical PMS, a condition characterized by irritability, tension, depressed mood, tearfulness, and mood swings at specific times of the month. Symptoms are often mild, but sometimes they can be severe enough to affect daily activities substantially.

THE ADULT FEMALE BRAIN

As the adolescent years make way for adulthood, the brain continues to mature, and its streamlining process continues well into our twenties. The prefrontal cortex also further develops at this stage, a nod to twenty-one being the minimum legal age in the United States to purchase alcohol. Whether it's maintaining one's first credit line or keeping a plant alive for more than a few weeks, many of us find that we are now more capable than we thought and possess better judgment than ever before, as our brains master the ability to look ahead.

Women's brains in particular come into adulthood gifted with an excellent ability to recall specific aspects of verbal information, such as the precise details of a conversation, as well as episodic memory—the ability to recall details of past personal experiences, chiefly what, where, and when they happened. This fact may explain how so many women seem to possess crystal clear recall of conversations their husbands swear never occurred! All kidding aside, young adult women come equipped with a mature brain, a sharp memory, and fluent communication skills. At the same time, though, the internal processes that make and remake the brain (namely, the death and birth of neurons and their fluctuating activity) will rise and fall with each of our menstrual cycles, and throughout our lives. In fact, even once the brain has reached its mature state, it remains plastic, retaining the capacity to shift and change in response to our life experiences. These brain-body shifts are never more evident than . . . when a woman becomes pregnant.

Now, a word about pregnancy. Not all of us choose this path, I'm aware, instead directing our courage and magic elsewhere. I hope that each of us will be lauded for our signature shine in due course. For the purposes of this chapter, I speak to the potential of motherhood, a deeply unsung role that needs to garner the proper respect. To my mind, the most significant contribution that science can provide is to highlight how pregnancy and motherhood change the female brain in ways that, while rendering us vulnerable to some extent, release in us an as-yet-unrecognized resilience. Understanding that each of the Three P's carries both vulnerabilities and resilience is key to understanding and accepting not just menopause but womanhood as a whole.

HOW PREGNANCY CHANGES THE BRAIN

The journey of becoming a mother is undoubtedly one of the most monumental experiences a person—and a body—can have. A slew of changes occur, many immediately apparent: bellies are growing, breasts are as well, and morning sickness might disturb you far past noon. But all these changes belie an essential fact: bringing a new life into the world impacts your *brain* just as much as it does the rest of you. Once again, your hormones exert as powerful an influence on the inside as on the outside. Estrogen and progesterone rise enormously, ballooning fifteen to forty times beyond their usual levels. Oxytocin, affectionately coined the love hormone, enters the mix, too. And if you recall, the brain is involved in the making of all of these hormones and is impacted by them in return. As a result, a woman's brain may change more quickly and drastically during pregnancy and postpartum than at any other point in her life, including puberty. However, much like what happens in puberty, while your body is growing, your brain is downsizing.

Research demonstrates that pregnancy is marked by extensive *reductions* in the brain's gray matter. In the most comprehensive study so far, researchers did brain scans on twenty-five first-time mothers before they became pregnant and then again during the first few weeks after giving birth. Their gray matter had shrunk so consistently that a computer algorithm could predict with complete accuracy whether a woman had been pregnant just by looking at her brain!

The scientists were so puzzled by these findings that they decided to peek inside the workings of the moms' brains in a different way—by showing them pictures of their infants. The data showed a compelling revelation. Several of the same brain areas that had lost gray matter during pregnancy were the very ones that responded with the most boisterous brain activity to photos of the mom's own baby as opposed to photos of other infants. After all aspects of the data had been reviewed, it became clear that the more profound the decrease in gray matter during pregnancy, the stronger the bond between mom and baby after giving birth. As odd as these results may seem, there's a reasonable explanation. If we look at this from the brain's perspective, pregnancy isn't too dissimilar from puberty. Remember that during puberty, surges in sex hormones cause a loss of gray matter, as unnecessary brain connections are pruned, a process that sculpts the teen's brain into its adult form. This *loss* precipitates a *gain*: maturation. A teen's smaller brain simply reflects more streamlined brain circuitry. Scientists believe that pregnancy triggers a comparable development. As certain links between neurons drop away to encourage the formation of new, more valuable connections, the brain becomes leaner to get meaner all over again.

This is how I like to think about it: For those skills that have become second nature (doing basic math, cooking, driving), the brain no longer needs to hold the neuronal space to support them. This "automatic pilot" function allows the brain to dump what's superfluous and refurbish new mental pathways—those that will allow new moms to better respond to motherhood's myriad demands and urgencies. Sure enough, in the above study, another round of brain scans done two years after childbirth showed that the gray matter loss stuck around in some parts of the brain, but the hippocampus and amygdala had actually *grown back*, their size returning to pre-pregnancy levels. The frontal cortex also displayed a similar restoration. These regions' functionality was also off the charts. Take the amygdala in particular, which is involved in experiencing love and affection but also acts as a generator of the motivations and emotions that govern parental instincts, everything from nursing and protecting one's child to the impulse to engage and play with them. While the passage of puberty was about balancing instincts with rationality, pregnancy pivots us back toward our instincts instead, designating renewed space in which to activate them—and give them the credit they deserve.

The Supermom Brain

Though moms are rarely caught wearing star-spangled capes or wielding magic shields, one worth her salt rates superhero status in my book. As the days, weeks, and years roll on, many new mothers realize how quickly they acquire an impressive arsenal of skills many never knew existed pre-motherhood. These superpowers are not only near universal but scientifically proven. For starters, one of the first skills you develop as a new mom is a heightened sense of smell. No, we're not joking about dirty diapers here. According to the studies, almost 90 percent of new mothers can recognize their little ones *by scent* thanks to a primal connection our brains establish with our babies. Although you probably have not had to pick your baby out of a lineup while blindfolded, rest assured, you would actually be able to. Your brain knows what to do.

Let's move on to the "love spell." This magic is mom's new aptitude to release copious amounts of oxytocin, especially during nursing and skin-to-skin time. This huggy hormone prompts the uterus to contract during childbirth before teaming up with prolactin to cue breast milk production. At the same time, this boost in oxytocin has a strong effect on the brain's emotional centers, compelling a new mom to be smitten with her baby, and vice versa, in ways that words fail to describe. The surge in oxytocin combines with that in another hormone, called *vasopressin*, prompting a very primitive instinct called *maternal aggression* to kick in. This term refers to the "mama bear" behavior a mother manifests in defending her offspring against threats, which is powered by a brand-new "mama bear brain" that contains a virtual GPS for tracking and protecting the child at all times. We've all done it. There might be five other kids in the sandbox with a purple onesie on, but every mom has the uncanny ability to scan and spot her own purple-onesie-wearing tot in a matter of seconds and run to the rescue. We are also instilled with the adrenaline and wherewithal necessary to draw a line in the sand(box), if need be, completing our task with aplomb. The adrenaline rush, once again, starts in the brain.

The genius doesn't stop there. Perhaps the most important upgrade is that the brain regions impacted by pregnancy are involved in the theory of mind, just as with puberty. This is a mom-specific longer-term spinoff of what we were discussing above—a heightened ability to see and recognize other people's mental states, feelings, and nonverbal cues, anticipating needs and probable reactions. Whether it's interpreting a baby's body language or her various cries and coos, being able to understand what is going on in someone else's head, especially when there are no words, comes in handy. When these cognitive skill sets light up, we can better form attachments to others—a key to developing closeness with our child and within our family structure. As a most helpful add-on, many moms discover that they can quite literally read minds via a sixth sense. Moms *just know* when something bad might be going down with their child because they *just feel* something isn't right—a combination of maternal instincts, a motherly spidey sense, and being around each other so much. Moms notice things they'd never pick up on in any other human—to the point that they can often predict their children's needs before tears flow or a fever breaks.

Motherhood is certainly among the most complex and demanding set of circumstances one can experience in life. Not only do our bodies need to go through a metamorphosis to grow and nurture a new human, but so do our priorities and day-to-day lives. Our brains intuitively, or more likely by design, understand this and alter themselves in the process. The good news is that pregnancy prompts brain changes that boost critical maternal instincts and conceivably strengthen social cognition skills simultaneously. The bad news is that the upgrade your brain just downloaded can come at a cost. The same brain morph that delivered shiny new features can also rearrange your memory and attention files, trigger changes in mood, and roll out a steep learning curve to our new operating system.

"Momnesia," the Baby Blues, and Postpartum Depression

The frowned-upon "mommy brain," aka "baby brain" or "momnesia," refers to a spacey, somewhat altered state where one may become more forgetful or scatterbrained. Whatever you call it, if you're a mother, you can probably relate. Combine equal parts hormonal changes and the extensive rewiring that is taking place inside your brain, plus a good dose of stress and sleep deprivation, and *boom*—over 80 percent of pregnant women perceive a decline in cognitive function. These changes persist postpartum, with almost half of all new mothers experiencing forgetfulness, a narrowed focus, and brain fog for months after giving birth. This makes sense considering that the mommy brain maintains its new, kid-centric architecture for at least two years post-birth. These sensations may cause new moms to feel that their brains aren't functioning as they were pre-baby.

Multiple studies indicate that some cognitive skills, memory first and foremost, can indeed be impacted by pregnancy and postpartum. Such functions include chiefly multitasking and "spatial memory" (the ability to recall where things are). For example, when you navigate your local grocery store each week, your spatial memory enables you to make a beeline to your favorite coffee without searching the entire store. However, if you find yourself having to do a double take as to where the coffee aisle even is, you can blame it on mommy brain.

What do we make of this?

First off, pregnant women and new moms aren't making stuff up. At some point, it's common to feel like your little bundle of joy has not only hijacked your body but taken off with your mind, too. So kudos for keeping your cool in the process. Second, and most important, these changes are temporary, effectively resolving over time. Third, studies have shown that even though many expectant women and new moms don't *feel* as mentally sharp as they used to, their IQ is unquestionably unaltered. As troubling as they might feel, these slipups manifest themselves mainly as minor memory lapses or brain fog, which can mess with our usual perception of ourselves but are in no way an illness. (Note how similar this experience is to perimenopausal brain fog.) For those who can't shake off the worry, there is *no* evidence these mental blips might be linked to a higher risk of dementia.

The foggy mental state associated with pregnancy and postpartum is likely a transitory trade-off for the new, highly specialized brain in bloom. Consider it sort of like growing pains. In effect, cognitive slips are likely a result of a change in priorities *at a neurological level*. Life is operating according to a new set of rules and requirements, and so are you and your brain. The fact that it can also be wonderful and rewarding doesn't render it any less challenging. Experts believe that the maternal brain becomes so intensely focused on the safety and needs of the child as to necessitate that other daily activities take a back seat. Forgetting to pick up milk or to put the laundry in the dryer is frustrating, but remembering 3:00 A.M. feedings and managing to mentally note and respond to the intricate web of a newborn's varying needs is *the* priority. More disconcerting is that fulfilling this new job description can go largely unnoticed, seen as expected or taken for granted— while not ticking off the boxes on the old list seems to garner more attention.

As a scientist and a mother, I find the idea almost laughable that new moms suffer from "reduced focus" or have "concentration deficits." Whether we are simultaneously cooking dinner and sending emails while holding a baby or driving and eating breakfast while mentally organizing the day's schedule, the circus act of being a mom forces us to do more than one thing at a time. As if that weren't enough, we do so with a frequency and a mastery that none of the standardized cognitive tests would ever manage to measure. So please take heart, these shifts are in service to a bigger picture, not ones that leave you wanting down the road.

Nonetheless, as another example of "no pain, no gain," pregnancy and postpartum are often accompanied by another challenge: mood changes. As many as 70 to 80 percent of all new moms experience some depressive symptoms within the first weeks to months after delivery. Symptoms commonly include mood swings, crying spells, anxiety, and difficulty sleeping. Interestingly, these mood swings can be similar to those of PMS—and even related to it, as women suffering from PMS before pregnancy are more likely to experience altered mood and depression during pregnancy. And women who experience mood swings during pregnancy are more likely to experience them again during menopause. This connection further reveals the underlying thread of hormonal continuity that spans a woman's life.

About one in every eight new moms will experience something more severe than the baby blues, struggling with postpartum depression. Postpartum depression is a medical condition characterized by major depressive episodes, deep sadness, sometimes crippling anxiety, and a loss of self-worth that can last several weeks or more. In the United States alone, half a million women suffer from this disorder every year. Sadly, postpartum depression has long carried a social stigma. Society has deemed but a single reaction acceptable in the face of motherhood, and that is joy. Any lack of joy has been met with radical disapproval. It is also expected that moms should show up equipped and proficient at their roles on day one. This messaging is not only unrealistic but misleading, putting undue pressure on the very person already carrying incomparable responsibilities.

Historically, mothers suffering from postpartum depression were called madwomen and even thought to be cursed by witches—or to be witches themselves. Quite remarkably, it wasn't until 1994 that the psychiatric community finally recognized postpartum depression as an actual medical condition. Three decades later, it has become a household term, and treatments are in place. However, many still don't believe this condition is real, filing it under "women's imaginary problems." To be clear, experiencing depression, moodiness, or anxiety after giving birth isn't in any way, shape, or form reflective of a character flaw or weakness. Mood changes are one of the many natural signs that your hormones and your brain are undergoing a transition.

Changes in biology notwithstanding, having a baby is as lofty a pursuit as they come—a quest that takes enormous strength of character to entertain, let alone bear up under and see through. Motherhood is easy and hard, beautiful and terrifying, and every woman's experience is sacred and important. In developing our children's brains and behaviors, we teach them the first lessons of love and seed their consciences. As society urges us to seek worth apart from and in addition to this calling, I hope mothers everywhere are aware of the worth of what they do and how far-reaching their touch is.

A TALE OF VULNERABILITY AND RESILIENCE

How does all this relate to perimenopause? Because when it comes to women's brains and the Three P's, every stage is marked by both vulnerability and resilience. Puberty, for one, is often remarked upon with an eye roll and a cringe. But while there is no question that this stage of life comes with its own challenges, we now know that the teen brain serves a higher purpose. The same brain changes that trigger mood swings and fiery emotions at the same time unlock intellectual and social maturation, helping teens learn how to manage the intensity of life, a precursor to navigating the rather weighty task of growing up and handling all that is ahead of them.

Pregnancy and postpartum are also stamped with the marks of vulnerability and resilience. Yet again, the mommy brain isn't just a state of distraction and weepiness, but rather an indication that our brain is developing vital new strengths and exceptional abilities. The changes our brains undergo serve a fundamental evolutionary purpose, preparing a woman for motherhood and, in doing so, supporting the survival of the entire species.

There are pros and cons—both are part of being born with ovaries and with a brain deeply connected to them. Keep this info handy because it will be a recurring theme as we explore the last of the Three P's.

7

The Upside of Menopause

A SHIFT IN PERSPECTIVE

As we've come to understand, our brains pass through a sequence of hormonal transitions throughout our lives, first with puberty and then with pregnancy, only to end in perimenopause. However, while a tsunami of hormonal power accompanies both puberty and pregnancy, when fertility recedes, many associate it with an ebbing tide instead—the beginning of the end. In both culture and medicine, menopause is stigmatized as a flat-out unfortunate event with little, if anything, positive to say about it. But this reveals only one side of the coin. Upon further examination, menopause is quite nuanced and much more individualized than sitcom stereotypes or medicalized portrayals would have us believe. Whether we're talking about information passed down from mother to daughter or directly from doctor to medical student to patient, the message has been flawed and sorely lacking.

One of the most obvious pitfalls is that until recently, neither culture nor science has bothered to perform a reality check on menopause. While they have harped on the downsides, the upsides have remained ignored. What's missing from the conversation, therefore, is an accurate understanding of how menopause fits into the larger picture of a woman's life. This understanding can be gained only by seeing menopause through the eyes of the women *living* it, in league with the latest scientific data. In exploring this life event without prejudice and free of preconceived notions, we discover that perimenopause is just one more stop along the ride, not dissimilar from puberty and pregnancy.

CONNECTING THE DOTS

Peering inside the brain, we see that the hormonal changes accompanying perimenopause trigger brain symptoms not too different from those of puberty and pregnancy. Changes in temperature, mood, sleep, libido, and cognitive performance are very common during all Three P's. As you can see from table 4, the similarities are striking. After all, they involve the same system, the neuroendocrine system, that gets activated and deactivated at different stages of our reproductive lives.

TABLE 4. Similarities Between the Three P's

	PUBERTY	PREGNANCY	PERIMENOPAUSE
Changes in body temperature	x	x	x
Changes in mood	x	x	x
Changes in sleep patterns	x	x	x
Changes in libido	x	x	x
Changes in memory and attention	x	x	x
Changes in brain gray matter	x	x	x
Changes in brain energy	x	x	x
Changes in brain connectivity	x	x	x

Let's talk about changes in body temperature, for example. Puberty may not be associated with hot flashes as we know them, but it sure comes with sweating—many times, lots of sweating—as the body's sweat glands become much more active at this stage. Additionally, for girls, body temperature changes slightly with every menstrual cycle, peaking with ovulation and falling with menstruation. During pregnancy, those same mechanisms can once again prompt an increase in body temperature (there's a bun in the oven, after all), which can sometimes morph into something else entirely: hot flashes. Although seldom cited, hot flashes are another symptom pregnancy and perimenopause have in common, with more than a third of all pregnant women sweating them out, too!

How about brain fog? It's a well-known fact that most teenagers have their heads in the clouds, with difficulty concentrating or remembering information. For girls, this can intensify during the late phase of the menstrual cycle. As we discussed, brain fog is quite common during pregnancy and postpartum, too.

What instead distinctly differs is how we perceive the first two P's versus the last. Puberty and pregnancy are no picnic either, but here we tend to focus on the positives. During our children's teen years, we fill photo albums with snapshots of them at the prom, on the athletic field, and in the classroom, celebrating a parade of coming-of-age milestones. We do the same with pregnancy, showering mothers-to-be with gifts and parties as we shop and prepare in anticipation of the baby's arrival. When hit with the tough stuff of these transitions, we stay upbeat. Whether it's pimples and periods or swollen ankles and morning sickness, we say to ourselves, *This, too, shall pass,* and tend to react with sympathy and support. If a teenage girl is irritable and has trouble focusing, we chalk it up to adolescence and give her time and space to muddle through. Similarly, if a pregnant woman is crying for no clear reason, we think, *It's her hormones,* and give her a hug. In both cases, we err on the side of optimism and encouragement. While this approach can inadvertently result in some serious symptoms not being addressed, the overall intention is one of allowance and reassurance.

But when those same behaviors crop up in a perimenopausal or postmenopausal woman, they are most often met with the opposite reaction: an absence of support, visible annoyance, or even disdain. Or at times, denial. Conversations about menopause lack, among so many other things, a nuanced language to help doctors gauge the problem in the first place. For instance, it is understood (and accepted) that some women menstruate every month without much discomfort, while others have a hard time, or PMS, or in more severe cases, premenstrual dysphoric disorder. Likewise, some women sail blissfully into motherhood, while others experience severe symptoms of postpartum depression, anxiety, and cognitive fatigue. The fact that we have words to describe this range of symptom severity not only enables accurate diagnosis and treatment but legitimizes their validity. There is no such distinction for women who experience severe symptoms of menopause. The compassion factor isn't there, either. During perimenopause in particular, many women are met with a sour "You still have your period, so grin and bear it."

It is no wonder menopause is felt as a moment of doom and gloom when those experiencing it are disregarded rather than embraced, the event itself interpreted as anything from sheer exaggeration on the one hand to a disease on the other. But the idea that menopause might put women at a disadvantage is one that history and culture—not biology—have inflicted upon us. In fact, from a biological perspective, some of the same *positives* that apply to puberty and pregnancy may well apply to perimenopause, too.

If you've been following how the prior two P's work, the fact that the brain changes during menopause (just like it does during those other milestone periods) won't be as surprising or alarming. So here's the million-dollar question: To what degree does menopause also deliver a customized update to your brain's operating system?

It is plausible that as the brain approaches menopause, it gets another chance to go leaner and meaner, discarding information and skills it no longer needs while growing new ones. For starters, some of the brain-ovary connections necessary to make babies are no longer needed, so arrivederci to that. But also all the neurologically expensive skills we reviewed in the last chapter—decoding baby talk, subduing temper tantrums, and high-level multitasking—are not as relevant once your birdie has flown the coop. They are still helpful, but not urgent. It only makes sense, then, that the brain would eventually start pruning away those expired connections—and what better biological clue to do so than menopause. Again, many believe that, as this latest and greatest brain update unfolds, that's when hot flashes, brain fog, and other bothersome symptoms kick in. Once the update is complete, the symptoms start dissipating (which may take longer than the other two P's because now we are . . . well, older).

All this information is helpful to place menopause under a much broader lens. But where are the bonuses? Could it be that the menopausal brain morph might better equip us for our later years? Could menopause come with its own ingenuity, proving instrumental in preparing women for a new role in life as in society? Despite society having turned a blind eye toward any menopausal perks, there is increasing evidence that this profound hormonal event also bestows new meaning and purpose on women.

HAPPINESS IS NOT A MYTH AFTER ALL

Any major life transition can be a chance at reawakening, even if the road is rough. While the general mindset in the Western world is that menopause takes things away from us, the untold story is that it's also busy endowing us with new gifts. Consider, for example, something everyone wants but few master: happiness.

You've heard that right. One of the more surprising things I've learned is that postmenopausal women are generally happier than younger ones—and generally happier than they themselves were *before* menopause. According to several studies, some of the most notable and overlooked upsides of menopause revolve around better mental health and greater contentment with life. In the Australian Women's Healthy Ageing Project, for example, postmenopausal women reported improved mood, more patience, less tension, and feeling less withdrawn as they entered their sixties and seventies. Similar results hail from studies conducted in Denmark, where postmenopausal women shared experiencing a stronger sense of well-being after menopause, with 62 percent stating that they felt, indeed, happy and satisfied. About half of these women also stated that they were as happy as they'd ever been, even at a younger age. Likewise, the Jubilee Women Study found that 65 percent of British postmenopausal women were happier than they were before menopause, feeling more independent and enjoying better relationships with partners and friends. If nothing else, these insights debunk the stereotype of the unhappy and dissatisfied postmenopausal woman.

Contrary to popular assumptions, preconceived notions, and even marketing, the evidence points to a fairly nuanced relationship between menopause and life satisfaction. Take a look at figure 8. The thicker line marks the effect of menopause on women's life satisfaction over time (with vertical lines marking differences among different women), starting five years before menopause through ten years after menopause. Time 0 marks the point when menopause took place.

Figure 8. Menopause vs. Life Satisfaction

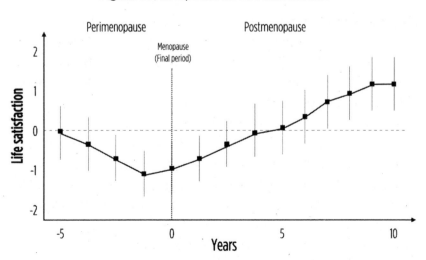

The most important data everyone needs to see:

- *Perimenopause*: Most women indeed grow unhappy in the three years or so building up to menopause.
- *After menopause*: Life satisfaction tends to remain low for two to three years after the final menstrual period, but then increases well past baseline and remains steadily higher over time.

The bottom line: Menopause tends to affect life satisfaction mainly *in the short run*. Most women adapt to the change, usually within a couple of years into their postmenopausal life. After this point, menopause no longer seems to have a negative impact on happiness and perhaps may even lead to more contentment. While this awaits confirmation, it is consistent with more general observations that happiness and life satisfaction tend to follow a U-shaped curve. Multiple studies indicate that contentment is relatively high in young adulthood but slowly drops and hits a low point at about age fifty (the average age of menopause). Then it steadily climbs to new heights later in life.[5] Believe it or not, by the time we're in our sixties, it's statistically probable that we'll never have been happier. Of course, everyone's different, and an individual's personal experience may stray from the norm for many reasons. Still, the U-shaped curve reinforces the notion that the midlife menopausal slump is *temporary*.

"Menostart": A Second Adulthood

Now, does menopause itself bring contentment, or are women happier after menopause because the symptoms are gone?

It just so happens that menopause can leverage a positive impact on your life in addition to its apparent hurdles. For one thing, not all its physical changes are negative. According to national surveys, the increase in mood and optimism reported by many postmenopausal women is often related to being finished with periods, PMS, and concerns about pregnancy. For many women, the end of their period is a cause for celebration in and of itself. It signifies the grand finale to certain elements of inconvenience: no more tampons, no more pads, no more cramps—after decades of them. Menopause also shrinks uterine fibroids, a major cause of heavy bleeding, and it kicks out PMS, which for 85 percent of women means the end of a range of complex symptoms from breast tenderness and irritability to debilitating migraines. This latitude is a big plus for more women than you may imagine. And as yet another positive note, enjoying sex without thinking about possible unanticipated outcomes is frequently cited as one of the utmost benefits of menopause.

But also, plenty of women have positive attitudes toward menopause—not only once the symptoms subside but even when they are in the thick of it. At some point in my research, I came across the term *menostart* as an alternative to *menopause*. This word seems apt for the many women who experience this life transition as a turning point, after which their interests, priorities, and attitudes shift in a positive way. A second adulthood, if you will, or a renaissance of sorts is entirely possible. American anthropologist Margaret Mead called it "menopausal zest"—the rush of physical and psychological energy some women experience after menopause. You may not have the frenetic energy of a teenager, but you may find yourself pondering new beginnings: a new career, new relationships and interests, new places to live or travel, renewed health and self-care practices, and an all-around refresh as to how you channel your time and energy. Many women are also only too happy to have more me-time as they wind down from full-time work and family responsibilities. While this is not necessarily thanks to menopause itself, the prospect of personal growth and the freedom to concentrate on their own interests is a luxury they are finally free to accept. As Oprah Winfrey once said: "So many women I've talked to see menopause as a blessing. I've discovered that this is your moment to reinvent yourself after years of focusing on the needs of everyone else." In the grand scheme of things, if that isn't a plus, I don't know what is.

Emotional Mastery

Hand in hand with contentment comes another much-coveted attribute: self-transcendence. Or, as some may put it, "giving fewer f***s." This theme repeatedly surfaces in postmenopausal women's accounts of their experience of this milestone. They describe the ability to draw a line regarding others' needs, finally able to pay attention to their own. Once they have managed menopause, whether it's been a stroll in the park or a walk through fire, many women tend to emerge more confident and less constrained, with renewed vigor and a take-no-baloney attitude.

During this period, some things take a hike, like the weight of pressures felt by youth, a preoccupation with various social games, or any inclination to wear Daisy Dukes. At the same time, new perspectives arise—a refreshed sense of self and an awareness of new opportunities and choices. This empowerment is due partly to biological triggers and partly to the timing of menopause. With fifty-plus years of life experience under their belt, many postmenopausal women have developed a nice set of life skills, giving them a greater confidence they can handle whatever comes their way. By then, a woman has experienced her own array of challenges, losses, illnesses, and disappointments, and has better discerned who she is, what she wants, and what she prizes. She realizes she is stronger and more capable than she imagined, and is much less likely to spend time brooding over bad experiences, mistakes, and blunders.

Notably, many postmenopausal women also report that emotions like sadness and anger don't hold quite the same charge as they once did, while the capacity to sustain joy, wonder, and gratitude often increases. There is a neurological reason for these shifts. Among other things, all the rearrangements in the menopausal brain may result in yet another upgrade to some networks involved in the theory of mind. Only this time, the transition brings forth better *emotional control*. If you recall from the previous chapters, how we respond to emotionally charged situations depends partly on how we're wired in our brains.

Connections related to the emotion-processing amygdala versus the impulse-controlling prefrontal cortex can influence our approach. Puberty asks us to lean into the prefrontal cortex's rationale, whereas pregnancy attunes us to our instincts (while striking a balance between our emotions and our head). Now it's menopause's turn. This time around, we are about to fine-tune the emotional amygdala in a highly selective and precise way: it becomes less reactive to *negative* emotional stimulation! If you present postmenopausal and premenopausal women with negative and positive imagery and compare their brain activity, you'll notice that the postmenopausal amygdala is less responsive to emotionally unpleasant information. At the same time, postmenopausal women tend to activate their rational prefrontal cortex more than premenopausal women do. This result reinforces the idea that, after menopause, we have overall better control of our emotions, particularly our reactions to sad or upsetting ones. Isn't that a superpower in its own right?

Greater Empathy

This fresh research brings to light new notions of resilience, well-being, and emotional flexibility with regard to menopause. For instance, menopause has been linked to a boost in another skill related to the theory of mind: empathy. As it turns out, postmenopausal women are the ultimate empaths. According to a study of over 75,000 adults, women in their fifties show greater empathy than their male counterparts, being more likely not only to react emotionally to the experiences of others but also to try to understand how things looked from the other person's perspective.

Other studies found that a specific type of empathy called empathic concern or sympathy continues to increase as women age. This may be particularly the case when it comes to caring for . . . grandchildren. As we pointed out in chapter 6, scientists believe that the brain changes occurring with pregnancy may be advantageous later in life, when older women assume the role of caregivers. In a recent study, researchers tested this theory by using brain scans to explore grand-mothers' emotional reactions to others. To do so, they monitored brain activity across a group of grandmothers as they perused photos of their children and grandchildren—versus images of children they didn't know. (If you recall from the last chapter, this study is similar to the one researching pregnancy.) The results turned up interesting infor-mation about intergenerational bonding. When the grandmothers looked at pictures of their grandkids, the scientists witnessed brain activity in areas associated with emotional empathy—which is the ability to feel another person's feelings or to put oneself in another's shoes. But when the grandmothers looked at pictures of their children instead of grandchildren, their brain activity relocated to areas of the brain linked with another form of empathy, called cognitive empathy, instead. Cognitive empathy is more about understanding another's feelings on an intellectual level, focusing not only on *what* someone is feeling but on *why*. Interestingly, the more a grandmother was involved in the everyday caring for her grandchildren, the more activation she showed in *both* the emotional and the cognitive empathy zones.

You may have experienced this yourself, in a real-life way. If you have children, have you ever observed that your mother has a different relationship with them than she had with you when you were their age? Perhaps she appears more relaxed, easygoing, and demon-strative? The findings I'm referring to help explain why. As a mother, you are tasked with molding and guiding your children, often with achievement-oriented tasks and accomplishments in mind. Generally speaking, mothers do this under the substantial weight of caregiving responsibility and demands. This responsibility is no longer the case when you are a grandmother, though, as it's now your adult child's job to carry that burden. While they are sometimes blamed for spoiling their little ones, perhaps grandmothers are finally at liberty to respond with more yesses than noes—along with an extra helping of dessert! This broader, wiser view is built right into the brain of a grandmother, acting as a backup for her child while prioritizing the preciousness of unrestricted love.

Personally, what I like most about these findings is the view of women's responsibilities changing through our lifespan, whether one has biological children and grandchildren or doesn't. I am moved by how many of us fulfill multiple roles, often beyond blood ties—and how our brains appear to adjust and adapt to the current circumstances, at all ages and in all walks of life. In this spirit, in the next chapter we will spotlight how women's brains continue to kaleidoscope into fresh talents and strengths for a lifetime of use, as we delve into the *evolutionary significance* of menopause.

8

The Why of Menopause

MENOPAUSE: BY ACCIDENT OR DESIGN?

While the biology of menopause—the when and the what—are relatively well understood, the *why* has still not come clear. For anyone with ovaries, menopause is a fact of life, one we tend to either ignore or take for granted. In reality, menopause is a long-standing biological riddle, one that scientists haven't managed to explain fully. In fact, menopause appears to be at odds with evolution itself. From an evolutionary perspective, the whole point of life is to survive, procreate, and pass on our genes to the next generation. Menopause puts a stop to the transmission of a woman's genes, evolution's sole argument for female longevity. As postulated by Darwin, "If the main purpose of females is to propagate the species, then going through menopause many years before dying should be selected against, unless there are distinct advantages to it."

Well, we are not dead, are we? It is undeniable that there is something unique about human menopause. If we look out across the entire animal kingdom, most females do in fact die soon after they lose their ability to procreate. Even chimpanzees, our closest mammalian relatives, do not typically live past menopause. The few who make it are zoo captives who survive just a few years more. The only animal species known to outlive their fertility are certain whales, some Asian elephants, possibly some giraffes, and one insect, the Japanese aphid.

Anthropologists, evolutionary biologists, and geneticists have all been spinning their wheels over this. Until fairly recently, menopause was written off as the *unnatural* result of women's increased life expectancy, treated as the unfortunate upshot of our living well beyond what nature intended. One long-held view, the evolutionary mismatch hypothesis, insists that there is no benefit to menopause. They posit that modern medicine keeping us alive longer has unwittingly duped our genetic code, and that menopause is a fluke.

Not so fast. There is also reason to believe the exact opposite might be true. What if evolution isn't as misogynistic as those who conceived of it? Perhaps nature doesn't measure a woman's worth based on her ability to crank out as many children as humanly possible. If you start thinking outside the box, as one so often *must* do with women's health, an alternative hypothesis starts taking shape. What if evolutionary forces are still behind menopause, but this time, they favor women for once?

EVOLUTION'S SECRET HEROINES: GRANDMOTHERS

The view of menopause as an evolutionary *adaptation* instead of an evolutionary oversight was developed in 1957 by late ecologist George C. Williams. His idea didn't gain traction until much later, thanks to field data collected by Dr. Kristen Hawkes, a professor of anthropology at the University of Utah. Dr. Hawkes pulled a team together to extensively study the Hadza, a group of modern hunter-gatherers who have lived in northern Tanzania for thousands of years. Observing communities like the Hadza gave her a time-machine-like peek into how our early ancestors might have lived. Her research, however, didn't start with menopause, but with food.

A seed of an idea began to develop as Dr. Hawkes watched women of the tribe collecting vegetables. Often with younger children in tow, women young and old went on daily excursions to pick berries, wild fruit, and nutritious tubers. Suddenly it became clear that these female foragers were providing the majority of calories and sustenance to their families and tribe mates. In fact, while the men went out hunting daily, they returned with a substantial haul only about 3 percent of the time. So dad wasn't bringing home the bacon, after all—mom was. But the researchers' work was further enlightened by a shift observed as the younger women went on to have children. A pattern quickly emerged that revealed coalitions of grandmothers covering all gathering and feeding responsibilities. Since then, many studies of modern hunter-gatherers have shown that grandma is doing much of the work the world over. Although these women are no longer *reproductive*, they remain markedly *productive* in providing food and carrying out the chores that keep a village running. By doing so, the grandmothers were at the heart of keeping their people safe not only by ensuring their food supply was secured and abundant, but also by maximizing reproduction potential and the passing on of genes so precious to human evolution. How so?

The idea is that prehistoric mothers faced a conflict between foraging for food for themselves and their families and caring for their new infants. However, struggling with this sacrifice was no longer necessary once grandmothers stepped in to save the day. As the elder women took over the care of their grandchildren, they also allowed their daughters to produce additional offspring, doubling down on the odds of survival of the species. Evidence of *just how much* impact grandmothers' contributions had on childhood survival led Dr. Hawkes to reevaluate what was known about menopause and human evolution. Her aptly named *grandmother hypothesis* proposes that ceasing reproduction around age fifty, and living to tell the tale, allowed older women to devote care and resources to their children's children rather than birthing and nurturing new ones themselves. Since the process of childbirth becomes riskier with age, this seems like it might be nature's way of leveraging a savvy bet. After all, grandmothers still ensured the survival of their genes, genes that were just two generations down the family tree. Notably, if it weren't for menopause, such contributions would be impossible. Suddenly this so-called anomaly could be seen as nothing less than the epitome of nature's wisdom.

Is Menopause the Key to Human Longevity?

The potential of nature taking menopause's side doesn't end there. Other evidence points to the idea that menopause may even be why humans evolved to live as long as we do today. In fact, the prehistorical grandmothers in question weren't just *any* grandmothers. We are talking about "naturally selected" grandmothers. Natural selection refers to the survival of the fittest. These women had the strength to survive childbirth multiple times *and* the genetic makeup to live past menopause, which, the theory goes, was bestowed onto their children and grandchildren, carrying grandma's longevity genes well into the future. Over time, this survival boost could have provoked an evolutionary shift, favoring and selecting for women who survived long past menopause. Under this hypothesis, postmenopausal life would become more and more common until, over time, every female *Homo sapiens* carried DNA with a cap on fertility *and* increased longevity in its place.

The theory is plausible, but is it scientifically sound?

Many believe so. For instance, research on killer whales, who also live past menopause, supports the grandmother hypothesis. Killer whale societies are matriarchal, and sons and daughters live out their lifetimes with their mothers rather than with their fathers. In addition, once mothers become grandmothers, they stick close by to help raise their grandchildren. In their world, it is indeed advantageous for mothers to lose their fertility after a certain age, eliminating any reproductive competition with their daughters and daughters-in-law. Match that with recent studies indicating how grandmother whales increase their aquatic grandkids' survival in other ways—for example, by sourcing food—and we begin to establish a pattern. Given that a similar societal pattern is indicated in ancient hunter-gatherer societies, perhaps menopause was nature's way of avoiding a similar mother-daughter conflict in our species, too. As we're about to prove, grandma's tendency to keep her kids' bellies full has long been part of human history—from as far back as our Paleolithic communities to our current-day holiday tables.

Grandma Lays the Groundwork

Baby chimpanzees, bonobos, orangutans, and gorillas are all cared for exclusively by their mothers. These primate moms are extremely protective of their babies, sometimes not letting other apes touch them for months after birth. In contrast, it's likely that grandmothers were present for their prehistoric grandchildren from the moment of birth. Scientists believe that it was common for children to be fed and raised by their grandmothers, so this bond likely fostered our species' deep social orientation. As humans, we distinguish ourselves from other animals by being able to sense the thoughts and intentions of others (the theory of mind) and to care about them (empathy). Both skills women in general, and postmenopausal women in particular, excel at.

Our ancestral grandmothers may have had a central role in building these senses. Think of it this way. If successful interactions with a child's grandmother made the difference between getting a full meal or going hungry, successful connection and communication between the two might also have bred critical social skills in the grandchildren. We still see modernized signs of this today. Images of grandma walking in the door are often punctuated by her grandchild's greeting her with outstretched arms and broad smiles, and the two embracing and exchanging a trinket or a sweet. At the beginning of our long history, this primal interaction may have begun with our bonding over tubers and berries. Whatever the case, caring for and feeding our young plays a critical role in promoting cooperation and social orientation in ways distinctive to our species. Our ability to figure things out by "putting our heads together" ultimately sets our species apart from all other animals. According to the latest research, a new picture of human society emerges, with fathers out hunting and mothers busy giving birth and nursing—while grandmothers kept the communal cogs oiled and rolling. It seems possible, if not probable, that humanity's evolution may have been built upon such a pattern, resulting in the unique timing of menopause and female longevity we see today.

WOMEN OF ALL AGES

Although everyone agrees grandmothers can provide welcome childcare support and resources for their children raising new babies, the notion that grandmothers were also integral in bestowing our longevity has been challenged. While scientists work it out, it's heartwarming to think of older women as evolutionary heroines, especially in light of the alternative narrative. The commonly held viewpoint to date is that postmenopausal women are a sort of collateral damage resulting from evolution's failure to sustain fertility throughout a woman's entire life. Are we satisfied with this explanation?

Once again, it is helpful to look at menopause through a neuroscientist's lens. Humans evolved under different evolutionary pressures than other animal species, pushing the development of distinctive cognitive and social skills. As we've reviewed over these past chapters, at various crossroads in a woman's life, brain-hormone events promote social and cognitive upgrades or adaptive advantages. Whether preparing us for adulthood after puberty, promoting nurturing abilities after pregnancy, or honing us for unique societal roles after menopause, our neuroendocrine networks seem to have a plan *in mind*.

The grandmother hypothesis may be controversial, but the importance of grandmothers in the lives of many families is not, and neither is the influence and benefaction of elder women in countless societies the world over. Grandmother by blood or choice, those that care for us in this way are of inestimable value and have been for millennia. Those who have known the blessing of one understand this implicitly. Since women today live far longer than ever, the time has come to roll up our sleeves and figure out how we can protect and invigorate our minds to ensure this legacy. While hormones may ebb, we shall not.

PART 3

HORMONAL AND NONHORMONAL THERAPIES

9

Estrogen Therapy for Menopause

THE ESTROGEN DILEMMA

What is it about hormone therapy that makes it so confusing? Is hormone replacement as dangerous as some people say it is—or is it the cure-all that its superfans insist? No matter how straightforward you wish the answer to this question was, it remains stubbornly layered with so many ifs, ands, and buts.

Unfortunately, this wild-goose chase is par for the course when we are attempting to make heads or tails of hormone replacement therapy, or HRT.* By the time a woman begins navigating menopause, HRT has undoubtedly crossed her radar. The idea behind this therapy is to replace those hormones that the ovaries cease to produce, chiefly estrogen (or estrogen and progesterone), with the same hormones contained in pills, patches, and creams, among other options. While this is logical in principle, weighing the benefits and risks has made this choice challenging for providers and patients alike. Many women are frightened of hormones due to warnings about increased risks of cancer,

---

* HRT is now referred to as menopause hormone treatment, or MHT. We shall stick with HRT, as most women are more familiar with this term.

heart disease, and stroke. Others are discouraged from going on HRT by their own doctors without further discussion. Others remain unclear about whether HRT can effectively treat menopausal symptoms in the first place, scouring the internet and discussing options ad nauseam with friends. Before long, however, confusion reigns and you find yourself on Amazon, perusing concoctions from rare jungle herbs that are supposed to cool your hot flashes and stoke your libido at the same time! We can do better than this.

This chapter aims to take some of the mystery out of the debate by reviewing HRT's actual bottom-line risks and benefits. We will first examine how HRT got such a bad reputation, and then explore the recent shift that has sparked a renaissance in the use of hormone therapy for treatment of menopausal symptoms, with a particular focus on the brain symptoms we've reviewed so far.

THE GOLDEN AGE OF HRT

In the past, menopause treatment was a veritable house of horrors, from opium to exorcism and institutionalization. Eventually scientists discovered estrogen and some of its functions, leading to the widespread use of estrogen replacement for menopause. In 1942, the U.S. Food and Drug Administration approved the first hormone replacement therapy drug called Premarin, marketed by Wyeth Pharmaceuticals (now owned by Pfizer). This estrogen pill quickly became a national bestseller.

Despite its meteoric rise in the seventies, at this point HRT hit the first of many speed bumps. It turned out that Premarin increased the risk of endometrial cancer in the uterus. However, researchers found that reducing the dose of estrogen and adding a progestin (a synthetic form of progesterone) protected the uterus, leading to the release of a second pill called Prempro, containing both estrogen and progesterone. The scare over, HRT was hot again. By 1992, Premarin was the number one prescribed drug in the United States, with sales exceeding

$1 billion. Millions of women jumped on the bandwagon, partly because Wyeth's marketing promoted hormone replacement as the ticket to a vibrant, sexy postmenopausal life, and partly because most physicians were also on board, suggesting it to patients without hesitation. Once women start losing estrogen, they argued, taking replacement hormones could cure hot flashes, protect against heart disease, keep bones strong, and improve one's sex life to boot—what more could a girl want? By this time, major professional societies were also endorsing HRT as an effective first-line solution not only for hot flashes but for the prevention of heart disease and osteoporosis. After all, early scientific studies and lots of anecdotal evidence backed up the claims: women on HRT reported having fewer hot flashes while also experiencing less bone loss and a lower rate of heart disease than those opting out. While HRT carried a risk of breast cancer that was worth considering, women were advised not to worry too much about that, unless a history of breast cancer was present. The choice seemed obvious: as soon as menopause hit, it was time to go on hormones. So by the nineties, hormone therapy wasn't just about being "feminine forever." Now it was also touted as "healthy forever."

The Fall from Grace

In 2002, a bombshell exploded in the medical establishment. The study at the center of the commotion was called the Women's Health Initiative (WHI). It was a federally financed examination of HRT started in the early nineties, extraordinary in both its scale and ambition: almost 160,000 postmenopausal women were enrolled in a multiyear comparison of estrogen pills with or without progesterone versus placebos. The goal was to provide conclusive evidence as to whether all this widescale prescribing of HRT was indeed a sound idea, with a particular focus on preventing heart disease. But on July 9, 2002, WHI investigators made the shocking announcement that they were pulling the plug on the trial *three years earlier than planned*.

As it turned out, HRT was "too dangerous" to the participants' health to proceed. The women on hormones had more heart trouble than their placebo-taking counterparts, instead of less. Their risk for stroke was on the rise, too, as was their risk for blood clots and breast cancer. Just as surprisingly, even their risk of dementia had gone up. Somehow HRT was doing precisely the opposite of what was intended and then some. The WHI bulletins dominated medical news all summer and long into the autumn. So dire were their broadscale warnings that millions of women stopped HRT on the spot. Sales of estrogen pills plummeted. Drug development for menopause came to a screeching halt. The news was out: HRT was now considered deadly.

THE WHI REVISITED: THE WRONG DRUGS, TESTED ON THE WRONG POPULATION

Over twenty years have passed since the WHI kaboom. A ferocious hormone debate has been roaring since, questioning both the study's validity and its findings. Now that the smoke has cleared, we find that the fine (and not so fine) print on the subject matters a very great deal.

The Importance of Having (or Not Having) a Uterus

Let's start with the basics. If you possess a uterus, then you will receive both estrogen and a progestogen (a generic term including different types of progestogenic preparations). (Just as a reminder, this is because estrogen alone can increase the risk of uterine cancer, while progesterone lowers this risk.) This two-hormone treatment is called estrogen-plus-progesterone therapy, but also combination therapy, or opposed therapy. If you've had a hysterectomy and no longer have a uterus, then you are not at risk for uterine cancer and don't usually need the progesterone. In this case, it is standard practice to prescribe estrogen alone. This is called estrogen-only, or unopposed, therapy.

The WHI study did include two clinical trials designed to reflect this distinction. The first trial, which caused such a stir in 2002, was designed for women with uteruses, who were prescribed Prempro, the estrogen-plus-progesterone therapy. The progesterone used in this preparation is called a "progestin," which is a synthetic form of the hormone. The second trial involved women who had undergone hysterectomies and were given Premarin, the estrogen-only treatment. Each group was compared to a placebo group of women who did not receive hormones. In the end, both trials were shut down due to an increased risk of stroke and blood clots. However, the risk of breast cancer was increased only for women taking the estrogen-plus-progestin therapy. The estrogen-only treatment had precisely the opposite effect, with a 22 percent *reduced* occurrence of breast cancer. The media, however, zoomed in on the cancer scare of the first trial, generating public panic around both types of HRT and leaving apprehension in its wake present to this day. Fortunately, we now have a more nuanced understanding of if and when this cancer risk exists, which we'll discuss ahead.

Oral, Transdermal, Bioidentical, Compounded . . . Oh, My!

Another fly in the WHI ointment was that different estrogen preparations can have different effects. Currently, there are two main types:

- *Conjugated equine estrogens.* The kind of estrogen used in the WHI trials is called *conjugated equine estrogen*, or CEE. CEEs are a concentrated formula manufactured from the urine of pregnant horses, which typically contains more than ten different forms of estrogen, mainly estrone, and smaller amounts of estradiol.
- *Estradiol.* Today, estradiol itself is available, and is called *micronized estradiol.* It typically comes from yam whose molecules have been tweaked until they are atom-for-atom identical to our ovary-produced estradiol. For this reason, it is also referred to as bioidentical, or body-identical estrogen.

Synthetic replications of the equine preparations, called *synthetic conjugated estrogens* (CE), are also available and so is synthetic estradiol (*ethinyl estradiol*), which is often used in hormonal contraceptives.

These are the main types of estrogen at our disposal. Additionally, the way estrogen is delivered and whether its effects are local or widespread also matters. HRT is a systemic therapy, which means it is designed to release hormones through the bloodstream to be absorbed throughout the body, therefore having systemic (whole-body) effects. This occurs via two main routes of delivery:

- *Oral route (by mouth)*. When the WHI was running its study, estrogen (specifically, CEEs) was taken at high doses and always orally, as pills. Oral estrogen metabolizes through the liver, possibly creating additional complications before going about its business. Scientists believe that the use of oral CEEs might have further muddied the waters of the WHI studies, as some studies have found that oral estradiol may be safer than oral CEEs.
- *Transdermal route (through the skin)*. Transdermal estrogen is absorbed through the skin and directly enters the bloodstream, bypassing the liver. Although clinical trials have yet to examine transdermal estrogen thoroughly, observational data suggest that it is less risky as compared to oral estrogen delivery. Transdermal estrogen is available via a skin patch, gel, cream, or spray.

Systemic HRT is different from local estrogen therapy, which is applied directly to the affected part and therefore has topical (local) effects. Low-dose estrogen preparations are used to treat vaginal symptoms of menopause, such as vaginal dryness, irritation, and pain. Topical estrogen is given in creams, suppositories, gels, or rings that are inserted directly into the vagina.

Estrogen preparations aren't the only piece of the puzzle requiring attention. It turns out that the type of progesterone can also make a difference. This can take the form of progestin, which is a synthetic form of the hormone, or progesterone itself, which is derived from natural sources. The progestin used in the WHI trials is called MPA (*medroxyprogesterone acetate*), and it has a problematic backstory of its own. Although MPA had the uterine cancer risk covered, there's reason to believe it may have been a factor in the higher risk of breast cancer. Now, this observation doesn't mean that MPA was the only factor at play. Nonetheless, newer preparations typically contain *micronized progesterone*, which, like the estradiol above, is a molecular replica of the progesterone women make naturally, making it bioidentical. Currently, there is little evidence that the combination of bioidentical estrogen and progesterone increases the risk of breast cancer. As a side note, while estrogen can be given in different ways, progesterone is typically given orally.

Before we move forward, I want to take a moment to clarify a few things about bioidentical hormones. The term *bioidentical* refers to hormones that are a perfect replica of those made by women's bodies. However, there are some claims that bioidentical hormones may be "safer" or more effective than other hormones. As long as we're talking about formulations that are FDA-approved and have been tested in rigorous clinical trials, other types of hormones are perfectly safe to use.

Another potential source of confusion is that both government-approved and compounded bioidentical hormones exist. In government-approved preparations, each ingredient is regulated and monitored for purity and efficacy, and tested for side effects. In contrast, compounded hormones prepared by a compounding pharmacy can use untested formulations and combine multiple hormones. They can also be administered in nonstandard or untested routes, and are sometimes prescribed based on salivary or urine hormone testing—a practice considered unreliable. Overall, the potential benefits of bioidentical hormones can be achieved using conventionally licensed products. Compounded bioidentical hormones may be a helpful alternative in case of allergies to ingredients in a government-approved formulation, or if specific dosages are not available. Now back to the WHI and, most important, how to use HRT to our advantage!

Timing Is Everything

Another major concern about the WHI study boiled down to timing. After years of investigating the investigation, we've come to recognize that the risks and benefits of HRT vary based on two other essential factors: a woman's age and the length of time she's been in menopause. This idea has been coined the timing hypothesis. In the simplest possible terms, estrogen's effects seem to depend upon when we start taking it.

In the confident kickoff of HRT decades before the WHI took place, most women went on hormones in their early fifties in response to menopausal symptoms. Contrary to this real-life usage, the vast majority of participants in the WHI were postmenopausal women in their sixties and seventies, if not older, and very few had any menopausal symptoms at all. This ten-to-twenty-year gap would produce a world of difference. In fact, many scientific studies have clarified that HRT works best while our bodies are still receptive to estrogen. This receptivity occurs when a woman is in the thick of menopause, and may extend as long as symptoms persist, but not long after that period. During this critical menopausal window, estrogen can improve and protect cellular health throughout the entire body. However, if given long afterward, estrogen may no longer have the power to strengthen or repair, but it may potentially cause detrimental effects. This fact clarifies how HRT could benefit a woman in her fifties while having no effects on or even harming a woman twenty years her senior.

Another factor worth considering: Given the age of the majority of women in the WHI study, many might have already developed some of the conditions the trial was looking to prevent. For example, since women's arteries have a higher propensity to harden after menopause, starting HRT late in the game might have made hormone therapy less capable of reversing or alleviating that problem. Since HRT also increases the risk of blood clots and older women are more susceptible to blood clots to start with, adding HRT into the mix may have contributed to the higher occurrence of heart attacks. Similar concerns have been raised regarding the increased risks of breast cancer and dementia.

Why, you might ask, would the most prominent drug trial in the history of women's health select women already long past menopause?

First off, when the WHI launched, precious little research had been done to clarify how estrogen actually worked in a woman's body and brain. If you recall from chapter 2, these mechanisms were discovered a few years after the WHI began. The timing hypothesis discussed above was formulated a full decade later. So the WHI investigators were missing some very important pieces of information. Additionally, as often happens in research, the decision to enroll women in their sixties and older was made on the basis of statistical considerations. The WHI was primarily designed to test HRT for prevention of heart disease, but the trial was scheduled to run for only eight to nine years. Since heart attacks and strokes tend to make their appearance after menopause, the only way the WHI could determine whether HRT could prevent those issues was by enrolling women already old enough to reach that danger zone before the study's time ran out. Unfortunately, that plan backfired.

The decision to use oral CEEs and MPA as the only test hormones was instead based in part on the limited HRT options back then and in part due to financial considerations. Drug trials are expensive. Wyeth offered to provide HRT free of charge for the entire trial, which was quite a deal. Besides, those same hormones were already being used by millions of women, so it made sense to test them in rigorous trials. And thank goodness they did. Although this was not the WHI's intention, the study revealed something highly critical: putting older postmenopausal women on pills containing high doses of oral CEEs and MPA (which was fairly standard back then) was not a great idea.

These facts should have constituted the leads in the newspaper articles instead of what most women heard on the news back in 2002. Further, dozens of studies since then have provided reassurance that for healthy women experiencing the symptoms of menopause, the benefits of taking hormones—given at lower doses and often via the transdermal route—generally outweigh the risks. However, these findings have trickled in, with no one story gaining the same kind of exposure or momentum as reporting on the WHI did. As a result, HRT's reputation has never fully recovered, and the consequences have been wide-reaching. With the old study still ringing in our heads, most women remain understandably conflicted about whether to use HRT for relief of their menopausal symptoms.

THE WINDOW OF OPPORTUNITY

If we've discovered there's a time beyond which it's best to avoid HRT, what about when to start it? Is HRT safer for women *younger* than those studied in the WHI—perimenopausal women and postmenopausal women who still have symptoms, which is a sign that your body and brain are still transitioning?

Today, the timing hypothesis is picking up steam. Scores of scientific studies have shown that HRT started at the right time can lessen the symptoms of menopause while also potentially protect against heart disease and other chronic conditions. For instance, studies of monkeys have shown that estrogen can be a strong protectant against heart disease when it's given during monkey menopause. When estrogen is administered to primates the equivalent of six human years after this period, it offers no protective effect—the window has passed. Scientists using mice to find a cure for Alzheimer's disease are discovering a similar pattern. When estrogen is given to perimenopausal or recently postmenopausal mice, it spurs cell growth, supports brain function, and can even prevent the formation of Alzheimer's plaques. But when given too long after menopause, HRT provides no benefit and may be harmful to the animals instead.

Overall, several lines of evidence suggest that HRT might be beneficial against these conditions when started early. For instance, the WHI did include a small percentage of women who were in their fifties, or more generally within ten years of the onset of menopause, when the studies began. For those women, HRT was associated with a *reduced* risk of heart attacks and deaths from heart disease and an overall lower mortality rate than those who did not take hormones. There is also emerging evidence that HRT may protect against cognitive decline, at least for some women, an issue we'll discuss in greater detail later. Thankfully, a growing number of positive observations such as these have led to a change of heart about how to use HRT for clinical practice.

Updated Guidelines for HRT Use

Until recently, most professional societies recommended *extreme* caution when taking HRT. Women were advised to use HRT for a limited number of symptoms, at the lowest possible dose, and for the shortest amount of time. Then in 2022, after thorough review of many positive findings that had accumulated over time, the North American Menopause Society published an updated position statement including striking revisions about the risks and benefits of HRT. These revisions, which have been endorsed by another twenty international organizations, grant more flexibility while also taking into consideration that every woman is different. Let's review these important updates.

Is HRT a Breast Cancer Risk?

The number one question for every woman approaching menopause is whether estrogen replacement will increase their breast cancer risk. Do I go on hormones and get rid of the hot flashes but risk cancer—or pass on HRT, soldier on, and hope that eventually the symptoms go away?

As we've discussed, these concerns were instigated by the WHI results; specifically, the 26 percent increased risk of breast cancer observed with the estrogen-plus-progestin formulation. Once again, let's return to the fine print. Out of the entire cohort, 38 women taking HRT developed breast cancer, compared to 30 in the placebo group. If you do some simple math, that's 26 percent more cases. However, in actual numbers, taking HRT resulted in only 8 more cases of breast cancer in total. So another way to think about this is that for every 10,000 women taking hormones (i.e., that specific combination of oral CEE plus progestin), an additional 8 developed breast cancer. These are much less striking odds than implied by a 26 percent increased risk.

Another thing worth considering is that the increase in breast cancer risk emerged only after five years of treatment—and twenty years later, the mortality rate of women taking hormones was no higher than that of the placebo group. And let's not forget about the other WHI trial, in which the estrogen-only treatment for women with hysterectomies resulted in 7 *fewer* breast cancer cases than placebo—that's a 24 percent *reduction*. These are important nuances we don't hear about enough.

Based on these and additional data collected after the WHI ended, most professional societies now agree that the overall risk of breast cancer related to HRT is in fact low, with current guidelines defining it as a "rare occurrence." In the words of Dr. JoAnn Pinkerton, executive director of the North American Menopause Society, "Most healthy women under age 60 or within ten years of having their last period can take hormone therapy without fear if taking estrogen alone or combined with progesterone."* When started within this time frame, HRT can be helpful to alleviate many symptoms of menopause, and it has been associated with a reduced risk of hip fracture, heart disease, colorectal cancer, and diabetes mellitus in the long term, too. A caveat here: This is contingent upon there being no previous history of breast cancer, as the risk of cancer reoccurrence remains a concern. If this is an urgent concern, skip to chapter 11, which is specifically focused on this topic. For cancer-free women, let's look at some numbers:

---

* https://www.sciencedaily.com/releases/2022/08/220824152312.htm

- Estrogen-plus-progesterone therapy does not significantly increase the risk of breast cancer in the short term (less than five years), but it is associated with a relatively small increase in risk over the long term (over five years). This increase is more closely associated with oral CEEs combined with MPA (the synthetic form of progesterone used in the WHI) than newer formulations, such as bioidentical estrogen and progesterone.
- Estrogen-only therapy does not increase the risk of breast cancer for cancer-free women without a uterus—that is to say, those who have had a hysterectomy—when taken for up to ten years. While we don't have enough definitive data after this ten-year window, observational studies suggest the risk of cancer may remain low for longer times.
- Vaginal (topical) estrogen has not been linked with an increased risk of breast cancer in the short or long term.

Another helpful thing to do is to put the risk of breast cancer associated with HRT into context. In fact, there are several common medical and lifestyle factors that pose a similar or greater risk of breast cancer compared to HRT. For example, simply leading a sedentary life carries a similar risk of breast cancer as HRT. But also, consuming two glasses of wine per day or carrying significant excess weight can double the risk of breast cancer compared to any form of HRT. Therefore, while the discussion around HRT and cancer risk is crucial, it's equally important to consider this within the larger picture of overall health, lifestyle, and medical choices.

Short-Term vs. Long-Term Use

For many years, professional guidelines stated that one should use the lowest dose of HRT for the shortest amount of time needed to keep the symptoms under control, and even then, only when indicated. The medical community now acknowledges that position may have been inadequate and even harmful for some women. Today, there is consensus that HRT does not need to be routinely discontinued in those older than sixty, especially in the presence of persistent menopausal symptoms or quality-of-life issues. According to professional societies, the data no longer support that cutoff and arbitrary limits should not be placed on the duration of treatment if symptoms persist, though an individualized reevaluation of risks and benefits is always recommended.

Spontaneous, Early, and Surgical Menopause

The biggest takeaway from the last two decades of research is that age matters. Contrary to popular knowledge, hormone therapy is actually recommended for women who go through menopause early, in the absence of contraindications. HRT can be beneficial for those with premature or early menopause resulting from genetic factors, primary ovarian insufficiency (POI), or autoimmune or metabolic disorders, and particularly in case of surgical menopause following oophorectomy. Surgical menopause is a far more challenging experience for most women compared to spontaneous menopause. Unfortunately, little thought or preparation is given to those undergoing this procedure, who are often left in the dark as to what happens afterward. So it's really important to underline that HRT is a viable choice for many women experiencing early menopause following oophorectomy. Experts believe that eligible patients should be encouraged to start HRT as soon as possible after surgery and to *stay* on HRT at least until the average age of menopause, approximately age fifty-one. This regimen has been shown to effectively treat hot flashes and vaginal discomfort, and to protect against bone loss. Observational data also show that estrogen therapy, along with progesterone if the uterus is present, may reduce the risk of future heart disease and cognitive impairment after oophorectomy.

Starting HRT After Menopause

What if you are over sixty years old or more than ten years past menopause? Is it safe to start HRT then? Considering everything we know and don't know from the research, this requires careful consideration. If there's one thing we've learned from the WHI, it is that starting high-dose oral estrogen long after menopause might increase the risk of some chronic conditions, such as heart disease. If HRT is to be started after age sixty or more than ten years past menopause, professional societies recommend low doses of hormones and preferably transdermal options like the patch or gel to alleviate persistent menopausal symptoms or quality-of-life issues. In the absence of rare contraindications, vaginal estrogen can be started at any age.

Contraindications vs. Approved Indications for HRT

Contraindications for systemic hormone therapy currently include:

Pregnancy

Unexplained or abnormal vaginal bleeding

Active liver disease

Uncontrolled hypertension (high blood pressure)

Known or suspected hormone-sensitive cancer, such as breast cancer

Current treatment for breast cancer

Active or recent arterial thromboembolic disease (that is to say, a blood clot that develops in an artery)

Previous or current venous thromboembolism (VTE; that is to say, blood clots in the veins, the legs, or the lungs)

Previous or current coronary heart disease or coronary artery disease, stroke, or myocardial infarction

There may, however, be exceptions based on personal medical history, which are important to discuss with your provider. For example, having had a blood clot is considered a "soft" contraindication that requires further evaluation. The route of HRT administration can also make a difference, as the risk of stroke and blood clots is lower with transdermal routes. Importantly, having a family history of any of the above conditions is not a contraindication, though it warrants medical review. To clarify this concept, hormones are not usually recommended if you *personally* have (or had) estrogen-dependent cancer—not because someone in your family has (or had) breast cancer.

For eligible women, HRT is not only recommended but FDA-approved for:

▶ VASOMOTOR SYMPTOMS

HRT remains the most effective first-line treatment for relief of moderate to severe vasomotor symptoms of menopause, aka hot flashes and night sweats. In clinical trials, both estrogen-alone and estrogen-plus-progesterone regimens reduced the number of hot flashes by about 75 percent while also reducing their intensity. Transdermal formulations seem to be as effective as oral options.

▶ PREVENTION OF OSTEOPOROSIS

HRT has been shown to prevent bone loss and reduce fractures in women without osteoporosis. If one already has osteoporosis, other medications are best.

▶ GENITOURINARY (GENITAL-URINARY) SYMPTOMS

The genitourinary syndrome of menopause (GSM) includes vaginal dryness, burning, and irritation, pain and diminished lubrication with sexual activity, as well as urinary incontinence, overactive bladder, and recurrent urinary tract infections (UTIs). The preferred treatment is low-dose vaginal estrogen dispensed as creams, tablets, rings, and soft gel vaginal inserts that you can apply to the vaginal area to reduce chafing, dryness, and tissue thinning. Regrettably, only 25 percent of women suffering from vaginal atrophy use this treatment, partly due to concerns around breast cancer. That's in part because of the FDA's inclusion of a black-box warning on the package label, which has further discouraged both doctors and patients from considering this option. However, these warnings are based on the findings of the WHI, which did not assess the use of vaginal estrogen at all. So, let me repeat this: low-dose vaginal estrogen has not been linked with an increased risk of cancer. In some rare cases, some patients may not be eligible for local estrogen, in which case the first-line treatment is a nonhormonal vaginal moisturizer. Note that vaginal estrogen may not increase libido or sexual interest. Systemic HRT is best in this case, and transdermal estrogen formulations may be preferred to oral. Testosterone therapy is another option, which we'll discuss in the next chapter.

Other Indications

Although HRT is not currently FDA-approved for changes in sleep, mood, or cognitive performance during menopause, many clinicians prescribe it based on reports of its beneficial effects, especially during the hormonal upheaval of the perimenopausal years. Specifically:

▶ SLEEP DISTURBANCES

Although more evidence is needed, several studies indicate that low-dose estrogen with or without progesterone may reduce sleep disturbances in perimenopausal women, in part by reducing night sweats, while also improving insomnia in postmenopausal women.

▶ DEPRESSIVE SYMPTOMS

In this case, it's important to first clarify whether the symptoms are a result of perimenopausal depression or major depression. Is it a hormonal response, or another underlying cause? The appropriate treatment will vary accordingly. Antidepressants or psychotherapy are the primary treatment for major depression, whereas estrogen therapy is the first-line treatment for mild depressive symptoms associated with perimenopause. It produces effects similar to antidepressant medications while also targeting the root cause of these symptoms. Estrogen therapy can be taken in combination with antidepressants if needed. However, estrogen therapy is not recommended for *severe* depressive symptoms, so it is important to consult with a qualified healthcare professional to make an informed decision. According to current guidelines, HRT may not be effective as a treatment for depression after menopause, although it may help improve the clinical response to antidepressants, especially for postmenopausal women who are still experiencing hot flashes.

▶ BRAIN FOG AND FORGETFULNESS

As is apparent, women's cognitive health is at the heart of my work, so of course I looked into HRT for memory support and dementia prevention. First off, can HRT conceivably improve the perimenopausal dip in cognitive function? The results are encouraging, as there is evidence that estrogen therapy started during perimenopause or early menopause can support and even enhance some aspects of cognition, primarily memory. While more rigorous research is needed, HRT seems to help with brain fog and forgetfulness, at least for some women. These beneficial effects are particularly evident for those undergoing hysterectomy or oophorectomy procedures.

The other big question is: Can HRT prevent dementia later in life? Unfortunately, the WHI remains the only clinical trial testing HRT effects for dementia prevention. As you know, those studies looked at women who were already postmenopausal by a long shot. Perhaps unsurprisingly, they showed no effects or even detrimental effects depending on the type of HRT used. The combination of oral CEEs plus MPA increased the risk of dementia when started in postmenopausal women in their late sixties or older. On the other hand, estrogen-alone therapy did not increase the risk of dementia relative to placebo, which is reassuring but still not the answer we're hoping for. Two important things to keep in mind are that we don't know whether other HRT formulations might yield different results and that the women to test are the ones *in the thick of* menopause, not those decades past it.

Unfortunately, clinical trials of younger women receiving HRT when the therapy is more likely to work, which is during the transition to menopause or soon after, are lacking. There hasn't been a single clinical trial of hormone therapy for dementia prevention among women in perimenopause, which is simply unacceptable. Nonetheless, reexaminations of the fewer younger women (those fifty to fifty-nine) included in the WHI provided important evidence that HRT started in midlife may indeed help to reduce the risk of dementia. Results show that, as these women got older, those taking estrogen in midlife didn't develop cognitive declines nearly as often as those given a placebo. Several observational studies report similar findings, prompting many clinicians to advocate for taking HRT during perimenopause or early menopause to sustain neurological health in older age. For now, in the absence of more definitive findings, HRT is not recommended to prevent or treat cognitive decline or dementia. While we're not there yet, I hope these recommendations will further shift and evolve as we gather more evidence.

The Next Generation of HRT: Designer Estrogens

When it comes to HRT, many feel like they have to take sides. Opt in or opt out? Take it or leave it? As the ping-pong match around this topic remains endless, women are effectively being asked to choose between their breasts and their brains. As a scientist, I believe we're asking the wrong question. We don't need to make do with quantifying trade-offs of what's currently available—we need better solutions. The question we should be asking is: Could we develop a type of HRT that is proven to support brain function *and* does not increase the risk of cancer? Sounds too simple or too good to be true?

Enter the new generation of so-called designer estrogens. This is to say, estrogens that are designed to do what women need. These compounds are called SERMs, which stands for selective estrogen receptor modulators. SERMs can block estrogen effects in certain parts of the body while acting like estrogen and potentiating its effects in other parts. By doing so, SERMs can offer many of estrogen's benefits without some of its possible risks. Many SERMs are available in clinical practice. For example, a SERM called tamoxifen is commonly used as a first-line treatment for breast cancer. Tamoxifen blocks estrogen receptors in breast tissue, effectively stopping estrogen from binding to cancer cells in the breast and making them grow. At the same time, however, it mimics estrogen effects in other parts of the body, like in the bones, where it may have positive effects. It's this ability to block estrogen in certain areas of the body while activating it in others that makes SERMs . . . selective.

After years of rigorous research, Dr. Roberta Diaz Brinton (my mentor and colleague) succeeded in developing a SERM *for the brain*. It is called PhytoSERM. *Phyto* means that the estrogen comes from plants. This genius formulation was developed to selectively supply estrogen to the brain, while being largely inactive or even inhibitory in reproductive tissue—that is to say, it does not increase the risk of breast or uterine cancer. You can think of PhytoSERM as a plant-based estrogen GPS for the brain: it bypasses the reproductive organs, making a beeline to deliver all the benefits of estrogen directly to the brain. In 2022, in collaboration with Dr. Brinton, we launched an NIH-sponsored, randomized, placebo-controlled clinical trial (read, a very thorough clinical trial) to test PhytoSERM for support of brain energy and cognitive function in perimenopausal and early menopausal women. This launch shows exciting promise. With clinical validation, we are hoping this estrogenic formulation will prove valuable not only to address the symptoms of menopause but also to provide extra protection for our brains, shielding them against dementia in particular. The trial results should be available around 2025, which, judging by how fast time is flying, is right around the corner.*

MAKING AN INFORMED DECISION

It is fair to say that menopausal women have been underserved—an oversight that should be considered one of the great blind spots of medicine. But as increasing research provides a more reliable picture of the

---

* I have no commercial interests in this work, and this is not a sales pitch. This is simply the announcement of the next phase of our research.

risks and benefits of HRT, things are looking a lot less grim than in the past twenty years. It's time to replace fear not only with knowledge but also with innovation. For many years, the decision of whether to take HRT was based on the one-size-fits-all approach of randomized clinical trials. It is now understood that each person needs customized attention, with continued evaluation of their own outcomes. Obviously breast cancer risk is an important factor to consider, but so are symptom control and quality of life—and every woman has not only different concerns but also different preferences and different levels of risk tolerance. There should be a holistic and individualized approach to managing menopause, perusing comprehensive, unbiased advice about the role of HRT as well as the full menu of lifestyle factors and nonhormonal remedies available to us.

For many women, the proper introduction of hormones can be nothing less than a godsend. But while it is necessary to modernize our understanding of HRT, it is just as important to underline that estrogen is not a magic bullet or miracle cure. While I totally understand the desire to offer HRT to women for whom it is indicated, the blanket use of HRT is not supported by science or the guidelines of the medical societies invested in menopause, and risks bringing us right back to the 1960s. There are many moving parts involved in working out the risks and rewards, and anyone who thinks there's a bumper-sticker answer to this question is neither listening to scientific argument nor reading the fine print. Estrogen can do many things—it can help with hot flashes, sleep disturbance due to hot flashes, low mood in early menopause, and osteoporosis prevention. Vaginal estrogen can help if sex is painful and for recurrent bladder infections. However, we need more research before HRT can be used for prevention or treatment of other medical conditions such as heart disease, severe depression, or dementia. Additionally, HRT simply doesn't work for everyone, no matter the type or dose.

Moreover, while it is important that we reevaluate HRT as a viable option for menopause care, women who are unable to take HRT due to medical conditions or side effects, those who don't require HRT, those who feel bad on it, and those who prefer not to take hormones may be feeling dismayed or left out. So I want to emphasize that respect for the diversity of women's health experiences and choices is extremely important. There is no one size fits all. All of us deserve to make our own choice armed with knowledge and options to do so. From nonhormonal prescription medications to lifestyle changes, there are other methods of managing menopausal symptoms, improving quality of life, and supporting overall brain health, which we'll discuss in the next pages. Remember, only you know what's right for *you*.

Other Hormonal and Nonhormonal Therapies

WEIGHING OUR OPTIONS

As we've explored the landscape of menopause throughout the last chapters, it's clear that one's experience of menopause is as unique as one's thumbprint. The methods of finding relief from its bothersome symptoms can be just as individualized. In recent years, the resurgence in HRT's popularity has brought comfort and relief to many women who experience menopause-related symptoms. However, although HRT may be the most well-known remedy, it's not the only game in town.

In this chapter, we'll delve into additional pharmaceutical options for treatment of menopausal symptoms. These include some hormonal therapies, such as testosterone therapy and birth control, as well as nonhormonal prescription medications. Nonhormonal management is an especially important possibility when hormones are not an option due to medical contraindications such as hormone-dependent cancers. In light of the recent emphasis on promoting HRT, cancer patients—who may already be coping with the physical and emotional stressors of their diagnosis and treatment—may feel excluded or as if they're being offered inferior options instead of the real deal. It is therefore important to underline that nonhormonal medications provide a solid alternative for managing menopausal symptoms. For example, paroxetine, an antidepressant medication, is approved by the U.S. Food and Drug Administration (FDA) for managing hot flashes. Other antidepressants, as well as medications like gabapentin and clonidine, also show evidence of efficacy in relieving menopausal symptoms. Just recently, in 2023, the FDA approved fezolinetant, a novel nonhormonal medication designed to treat moderate to severe hot flashes. Discussing all available options is essential to ensure that all women have access to appropriate and effective treatments for their own individual needs and circumstances.

Testosterone Therapy

As women enter menopause, hot flashes, mood swings, reduced energy, and low libido can crash the party, leaving many searching for relief. Enter testosterone, the hormone equivalent of a bouncer, ready to kick those pesky symptoms to the curb. But is testosterone really a reliable bodyguard?

While testosterone is typically regarded as a male hormone, women need it, too. In fact, our bodies produce three times as much testosterone as estrogen before menopause, in part because testosterone is needed to make estrogen in the first place. Testosterone is made by the ovaries, as well as by the adrenal glands and fatty tissue throughout the body. Because of this, its levels don't decline as much as estradiol levels do after menopause. Nonetheless, with aging, testosterone does decline, too, oftentimes taking sex drive along for the ride. Women with low testosterone levels may also experience symptoms of anxiety, irritability, depression, fatigue, memory changes, and insomnia. Additionally, while it is true that testosterone declines are typically due to the aging process rather than to spontaneous menopause, *induced* menopause can be associated with a much more abrupt loss of testosterone, which can be quite challenging. Women with primary ovarian insufficiency (POI) may also experience more severe reductions in testosterone levels. These differences are too often overlooked when evaluating treatment options.

Currently, the only clinical indication for prescribing testosterone is low libido. This is based on many studies and clinical trials showing that testosterone therapy can be effective to increase sexual desire, satisfaction, and pleasure after menopause. More often than not, HRT is enough to alleviate these concerns. However, if after a few months on HRT you are still experiencing loss of libido, as well as tiredness and fatigue, then it's worth having a conversation with your doctor about adding testosterone to your HRT regime. According to current guidelines, testosterone therapy in addition to HRT is considered appropriate if:

- You are postmenopausal, taking estrogen therapy, and have a decreased sex drive with no other identifiable causes.
- You have reduced sex drive, depression, and fatigue after surgically induced menopause, and estrogen therapy hasn't relieved your symptoms.

Although these guidelines don't specifically address perimenopause, there is no reason why younger women wouldn't benefit from testosterone therapy, too. This is particularly relevant considering that changes in libido often occur early in the course of the menopause transition.

Testosterone is currently not recommended to improve mood or cognition. Despite what you may have heard on the news, testosterone therapy for support of cognitive function in particular remains as controversial as pineapple on pizza. Here's why: While some studies have suggested that testosterone may have a positive impact on cognitive function, the available evidence is very limited. On the one hand, a few small-scale clinical trials have shown improvement in some aspects of cognition in postmenopausal women treated with testosterone as compared to those in a placebo-treated group. On the other hand, just as many small studies have reported no improvement. Studies examining testosterone's effects on mood in women are even more scant. In summary, we don't have enough evidence regarding these potential benefits to draw firm conclusions. As always, we need more research!

If you are interested in trying testosterone, here are three things to keep in mind. First, testosterone therapy for menopause typically involves administering a low dose of the hormone transdermally, through a patch, gel, or cream. Second, you don't need a blood test to decide whether testosterone is a good choice for you. That's because a low testosterone level in blood doesn't correlate with low libido or other symptoms. This also means that you don't need to start testosterone if your blood level is low. If you decide to start therapy, though, it may be helpful to check your testosterone levels over time to adjust treatment as needed. An annual review with your doctor is also recommended to look at symptom management and be informed about your own risks and benefits at any given time. Third, if you have libido-related concerns, many providers also recommend treating any vaginal dryness or discomfort with vaginal estrogen or other remedies. If there is pain with sex, it is recommended that you have your pelvic floor examined by a specialist and address any discomfort or pain before starting medications for libido.

Finally, while some women experience benefits from testosterone therapy, it is essential to carefully weigh the potential risks and benefits on a case-by-case basis. More rigorous work is also needed to provide clear evidence supporting testosterone therapy's long-term efficacy and safety, especially concerning its effects on breast and endometrial tissue. On the upside, testosterone therapy carries few side effects, chiefly an increase in body hair at the site of application. Contrary to popular belief, scalp hair loss, acne, and hirsutism are uncommon effects, as is deepening of the voice.

Birth Control

Another way to manage some menopausal symptoms may be a treatment you thought you were perhaps done with: birth control. While the primary purpose of contraceptives is to prevent pregnancy, hormonal birth control methods, such as combined oral contraceptives (COCs), progestin-only pills, and hormonal intrauterine devices (IUDs), all deliver small doses of estrogen and/or progesterone that can help regulate hormone levels, with balancing effects on the menstrual cycle. This can help reduce bleeding and menstrual cramps, and alleviate symptoms of conditions like polycystic ovary syndrome (PCOS) and endometriosis in turn. (Note: The intrauterine copper device, or IUCD, is hormone-free and not covered here.)

Here's how hormonal birth control can help during menopause:

- *Menstrual cycle regulation.* By providing a consistent supply of hormones, hormonal contraceptives can help regulate menstrual cycles and reduce the irregular bleeding experienced during perimenopause.
- *Hot flash reduction.* Clinical trials have shown that low-dose oral contraceptives can reduce the frequency and severity of hot flashes and night sweats. In several studies of perimenopausal women, those who received a low-dose oral contraceptive experienced an average 25 percent reduction in vasomotor symptoms.
- *Bone health.* Oral contraceptives taken during perimenopause can help increase bone density, reducing the risk of future osteoporosis.
- *Endometrial and ovarian cancer risk reduction.* Use of oral contraceptives has been associated with a reduced risk of developing endometrial and ovarian cancer.

Overall, hormonal birth control can offer some relief for women experiencing menopausal symptoms. As with any medication, it's important to consider potential side effects, health risks, and individual responses to treatment. Hormonal birth control may not be suitable for all women, particularly those with a history of blood clots, certain types of cancer, or other health conditions. Side effects can include weight gain, breast tenderness, and nausea. Mood swings and decreased libido are less common.

In recent years, there has been growing attention and controversy surrounding a potential link between birth control and mental health. This debate was fueled by a few studies reporting associations between hormonal contraceptives and an increased risk of depression. The largest study so far analyzed data from over one million Danish women aged fifteen to thirty-four, showing that those using hormonal contraception had a higher chance of starting antidepressants compared to those who didn't use hormonal contraception. These results made the headlines, prompting serious concerns. When we are looking at the data, however, it's important to note that the actual increase in the number of cases remained relatively small. In fact, about two to three women from the first group (hormonal contraception users) started using antidepressants every year as compared to one to two women from the second group (nonusers). So that's a difference of only one or two women. Nonetheless, women considering hormonal birth control should discuss their mental health history, especially a prior history of depression, and any related concerns with their healthcare provider in order to make informed decisions about their options.

Overall, hormonal contraception may be helpful as an alternative form of hormone therapy with contraceptive benefits during perimenopause, often providing a respite from vasomotor symptoms. If you are interested in this option, below are some frequently asked questions:

Will taking contraception delay or hasten perimenopause or the onset of menopause?

No, birth control neither delays nor precipitates menopause. What it can do, though, is conceal the menstrual irregularities that might have given you the first clues that you are nearing menopause. Combination pills (pills with estrogen and progesterone) cause a monthly withdrawal bleed that can appear the same as a monthly period. Even after menopause, you may continue to bleed similarly to how you would on your period. If instead you are using a progestogen-only contraceptive, such as the progestogen-only pill, implant, injection, or IUD, you might not have any periods at all. This can make it hard to tell if you've completed the transition to menopause. The best way to determine if you are in menopause while taking contraceptives is to receive an evaluation by an ob-gyn specialist.

Can HRT be used in place of contraception?

No, HRT is not a form of contraception.

Can you stop using contraception once perimenopausal or postmenopausal?

While the likelihood of conceiving drops after age forty-five, there is still a good chance. You can still ovulate (produce eggs) for as long as you are having periods, even if they are irregular. According to current guidelines, women under age fifty are advised to keep using contraception for two years after the last menstrual period to avoid pregnancy. Those over age fifty are advised to use contraception for one year after their last period. Your doctor can advise based on your personal situation and medical history.

Can birth control be taken together with HRT?

Many birth control methods can be safely taken along with HRT.

Antidepressants

While hormonal therapies can help with a wide variety of physical and brain symptoms of menopause, a well-informed conversation should also include a discussion of the role of antidepressants. In the realm of menopause management, antidepressants have garnered a somewhat negative reputation, primarily because women experiencing menopausal symptoms are often misdiagnosed with anxiety or depression. Consequently, they may be prescribed antidepressants instead of receiving targeted treatment for menopause. This misdiagnosis perpetuates the idea that antidepressants are an inadequate or inappropriate solution. However, when used correctly and under the guidance of a healthcare professional, these meds can provide significant relief from menopausal symptoms such as hot flashes and depression, while also improving the quality of life for many women. Specific antidepressants are in fact recommended as a first-line treatment for hot flashes in women who cannot take estrogen, such as those with hormone-dependent cancer. Importantly, many studies have been conducted in women with a history of breast cancer, indicating that these medications can reduce hot flashes by 20 to 60 percent compared to placebo.

It's also important to note that antidepressants may be just as helpful as HRT in specific circumstances, including treatment of severe depressive symptoms during perimenopause, treatment of depression after menopause, and treatment of major depression before or after menopause.

Antidepressants that have been tested for relief of menopausal symptoms include *selective serotonin reuptake inhibitors* (SSRIs) and *serotonin-norepinephrine uptake inhibitors* (SNRIs). The exact mechanism by which SSRIs and SNRIs alleviate hot flashes is not fully understood, but it is believed that their effects on serotonin and norepinephrine neurotransmitters play a role in regulating the body's temperature control. Currently, the SSRI paroxetine (the brand name is Brisdelle) is approved by the FDA for the treatment of moderate to severe menopausal hot flashes and night sweats. Low-dose paroxetine can significantly reduce the frequency and severity of hot flashes and night sweats, while also improving sleep, without negative effects on libido or weight gain.

Other antidepressants—citalopram (Celexa), escitalopram (Lexapro), venlafaxine (Effexor), and desvenlafaxine (Pristiq)—have also shown efficacy in menopausal women. In clinical trials, desvenlafaxine was shown to reduce hot flashes by 62 percent and to lessen their severity by 25 percent. Escitalopram reduced hot flash severity by about 50 percent. On the other hand, common antidepressants such as fluoxetine (Prozac) and sertraline (Zoloft) do not work as well for menopausal symptoms as the other antidepressants listed.

It's also worth noting that antidepressants can act quickly, usually providing relief within a few weeks of use. However, the effectiveness of these medications varies among individuals, and some patients might not experience significant relief or may experience side effects. The most common side effect is withdrawal symptoms. Additionally, some antidepressants, such as paroxetine, can interfere with tamoxifen, a common cancer drug, potentially reducing its effectiveness. Citalopram, escitalopram, and venlafaxine are safer options in this case.

Fezolinetant

Fezolinetant (marketed under the brand name Veozah) is a novel FDA-approved nonhormonal drug specifically designed for treatment of moderate to severe hot flashes. It is a type of medicine called a selective neurokinin-3 (NK3) receptor antagonist. This is because fezolinetant functions by targeting a protein known as neurokinin B that binds to NK3 receptors in the hypothalamus—the brain region that regulates body temperature. By blocking the attachment of the protein to the receptors, the drug alleviates the severity and frequency of hot flashes. Fezolinetant could be a game changer for women who are ineligible for HRT or those interested in alternative treatments. Its FDA approval also signifies an increasing acknowledgment of menopausal symptoms and the importance of addressing them, paving the way for more nonhormonal options to emerge in the near future.

From a practical standpoint, Fezolinetant is an oral pill taken once a day. Its safety and efficacy were evaluated in randomized, placebo-controlled Phase 3 clinical trials involving over two thousand women ages forty to sixty-five experiencing seven or more hot flashes per day. The results demonstrated a significant reduction in the frequency of moderate to severe hot flashes, by 48 percent for women taking a higher dose of the drug and by 36 percent in those on a lower dose, compared to 33 percent in the placebo group. However, as the trials lasted only one year, the long-term effects of this medication remain unknown. Fezolinetant has some side effects, including GI issues and elevated hepatic transaminases, which are a marker of potential liver damage. Therefore, it is recommended to undergo bloodwork before and during treatment to monitor liver function.

Gabapentin

Gabapentin (brand name Neurontin) is an FDA-approved drug for epilepsy that, in multiple trials, improved the frequency and severity of hot flashes and, perhaps more so, night sweats. Some feel that gabapentin may be a good choice for women experiencing menopause-related sleep disturbances because it promotes sleepiness. It may be taken as a single bedtime dose (if hot flashes are most bothersome at night) or during the daytime. Gabapentin can be taken with tamoxifen and aromatase inhibitors. Side effects may include dizziness, unsteadiness, and drowsiness, which typically improve after two weeks of use, and withdrawal symptoms.

Pregabalin

A close relative of gabapentin, pregabalin (Lyrica) is commonly used for seizures, pain, and fibromyalgia. It may help to relieve hot flashes, though it is less well studied than gabapentin in this regard. However, it can help reduce anxiety in menopause and can be taken with tamoxifen and aromatase inhibitors. Its side effects are similar to gabapentin but less noticeable.

Clonidine

Clonidine (Catapres) is a medication that lowers blood pressure and may be used to prevent migraines. It can be given to reduce menopausal hot flashes, though it seems less effective than antidepressants or gabapentin. It is also used less frequently than other medications because of possible adverse effects, including low blood pressure, headaches, dizziness, and sedative effects. Current guidelines do not recommend that clonidine be given before trying other options.

Oxybutynin

Oxybutynin is used to treat overactive bladder and urinary incontinence, but it can also help with hot flashes. It can be taken with cancer treatments such as tamoxifen and aromatase inhibitors. The most bothersome side effect is dry mouth.

11

Cancer Therapies and "Chemo Brain"

WORRIES ABOUT ESTROGEN AND BREAST CANCER

Cancer is a word that strikes fear into everybody's heart and can produce a deep sense of powerlessness. Few women are immune to worries about breast cancer in particular, the nightmare illness in nearly all calculations around hormone treatments. Most of us know someone who has had it or who is fighting it at present. If we haven't been touched by it directly, we are still well aware of the risk, in part because of other women's stories.

Every year, 1.4 million women worldwide are diagnosed with breast cancer, which still results in over 400,000 deaths annually. While breast cancer is a multifactorial disease, 60 to 80 percent of all cases are related to sex hormones. Many reproductive tumors contain so-called estrogen receptor positive cells, which are equipped with their own brand of receptors that attach to estrogen. As they latch on to the estrogen flowing in the bloodstream, they grow and get stronger. As a result, treatment for these types of cancer is aimed at blocking or suppressing estrogen to stop the cancer and then to prevent it from reoccurring. This can be done in combination with chemotherapy and sometimes surgery to remove breast tissue (*mastectomy*).

Two of the most frequently prescribed hormonal treatments for breast cancer, known as endocrine therapy in medical circles, are:

- *Selective estrogen receptor modulators (SERMs), aka estrogen blockers.* As the name implies, the job of estrogen blockers is to block estrogen receptors in cancer cells. They work like a broken key in a lock. By sticking to the receptors (the lock), they prevent the normal key (estrogen) from fitting anymore, thereby stopping the tumor in its tracks. The most commonly used drug is tamoxifen.
- *Aromatase inhibitors.* These drugs stop estrogen production in the entire body by obstructing the action of aromatase, the enzyme needed to produce estrogen. Aromatase inhibitors can be steroidal, like exemestane, and nonsteroidal, like anastrozole and letrozole. Without going into too much detail, this distinction highlights the different way these drugs turn off the aromatase enzyme.

These therapies can quite literally be lifesavers, often eradicating the disease completely or at the very least extending the life of millions of women. However, they affect estrogen action and production not only in breast tissue but in other parts of the body, too. Case in point: They can affect the ovaries, stopping ovulation and menstruation. This can be a temporary side effect or a permanent one—in the latter case, provoking medical menopause, no matter a woman's age. These drugs can also spur the telltale symptoms of menopause. For example, about 40 percent of women taking estrogen-blocking tamoxifen experience hot flashes. Other brain symptoms are also common, including brain fog and mood and memory changes, which many refer to as "chemo brain." These symptoms can be so severe as to make cancer patients wonder if they are experiencing an early onset of dementia. As you may have noticed, worry over the perception of one's diminished cognitive capacity to the point of fearing dementia is a common theme in this book, one that we seriously need to address.

In 2018, I wrote an op-ed in *The New York Times* about the connection between menopause and Alzheimer's disease. I did so with the intention of raising awareness about this pivotal life transition as an important yet largely overlooked element in women's brain health. I expected that it might stir up a number of strong reactions in various communities, but I wasn't expecting all the emails I received from breast cancer patients in particular. Because I highlighted the connection between a lack of estrogen and a possibly increased risk of Alzheimer's, many reach out still today, out of concern that their cancer medicines might be at unfortunate odds with the health of their brains.

Back when I was writing the op-ed, there wasn't quite enough data to answer these urgent questions. Thankfully, the past few years have seen an increasing awareness of the importance of estrogen for brain health—and it certainly helped that more and more women have been demanding accurate information about this important link and all its possible implications. All of this has spurred not only renewed interest in the topic but also more research focused on evaluating the impact of endocrine therapy on cognitive health in cancer patients, as well as fairly heated discussions on the possible role of HRT. It is this updated information that I am going to share in this chapter.

OVARIAN CANCER

Before we begin, it's important to talk about ovarian cancer, too. Ovarian cancer often goes hand in hand with breast cancer, in part due to the often undiscussed hormonal connection between our breasts and our ovaries. As with breast cancer, ovarian cancer becomes more common as women get older, the risk increasing after menopause. Our breasts and ovaries are also connected through a genetic component, as evidenced by the fact that some genetic mutations can increase the risk of both cancers, and the presence of one cancer can elevate the risk of the other.

Typically, treatment for ovarian cancer also involves a combination of chemotherapy and surgery, with oophorectomy being a first-line treatment. Oophorectomy can be unilateral (only one ovary is removed) or bilateral (both ovaries are removed). When the ovaries are removed along with the fallopian tubes, the procedure is called a bilateral salpingo-oophorectomy (BSO). BSO is of established benefit when ovarian cancer is found or suspected. It is also recommended in patients with significant family history of ovarian cancer or proven genetic predisposition, such as specific BRCA (BReast CAncer) gene mutations, and those with medical conditions known as Lynch syndrome and Peutz-Jeghers syndrome. However, there is accumulating evidence that ovarian cancer may actually originate in the fallopian tubes. Therefore, removing the tubes without the ovaries may be a viable strategy to reduce that risk for some individuals undergoing preventative treatment.

A downside of the BSO procedure performed before menopause is that it results in surgical menopause, which in combination with chemotherapy can make for an especially complex mind-body experience. This is important to be aware of, as patients are not always presented with a clear picture of what the long-term effects of these treatments may involve or of the courses of action available to deal with the symptoms that may occur.

CHEMO BRAIN IS REAL

Many cancer patients worry about or downright suffer from what they describe as mental cloudiness before, during, and after their cancer treatment. Sadly, chemo brain is another textbook example of how women's concerns around their cognitive and mental health have been dismissed by the medical field. Despite what cancer patients have been saying *for decades*, until very recently, physicians chalked up these symptoms to fatigue, depression, anxiety, and the stress of the cancer and treatment. The patients' belief that their symptoms were *not* due to being depressed, anxious, or fatigued was not taken seriously enough, either because some providers didn't believe that cancer treatment may have negative effects on the brain or because they lacked training to address these specific issues. Regrettably, many patients continue to encounter the same barriers even in the present day.

If you or anyone you know has encountered these issues, I am here to assure you that chemo brain is not just your imagination. *Chemo brain is real.* It is a *legitimate, diagnosable condition* that's receiving increasing validation and attention.

A main reason for greater acceptance of chemo brain as an actual medical condition is better imaging of the brain. Some imaging studies have found that chemo brain is associated with measurable changes to the brain's white matter, particularly to the fiber tracks connecting the hippocampus and prefrontal cortex. As you know, these areas of the brain are involved in memory and higher-level cognitive functioning. Other parts of the brain involved in cognitive functions can also undergo changes in both connectivity and activity following chemotherapy. These observations have significantly contributed to a shift in the general mindset by underscoring the direct impact of certain cancer therapies on the structure and functionality of the brain, thereby providing support to the reports of patients experiencing chemo brain.

Today, in the medical field, chemo brain is referred to as cancer-treatment-related cognitive impairment, cancer-related cognitive change, or post-chemotherapy cognitive impairment. I am not a fan of the word *impairment* in these phrases for reasons we'll discuss in a moment, but nonetheless, chemo brain is a symptom reported by as many as 75 percent of cancer patients. It is often described as difficulty processing information and feeling as if you can't think as quickly and as clearly as you did before you had cancer or started treatment. Everyday tasks require more concentration and take more time and effort to take care of. As you may have noticed, this is not too dissimilar from the brain fog experienced by women undergoing menopause. Here are some examples of what patients with chemo brain may experience:

- Problems with short-term memory; forgetting details like names, dates, and sometimes events; forgetting things that you usually have no trouble remembering (memory lapses); confusing dates and appointments
- Difficulty concentrating; reduced focus; a shorter attention span
- Feeling mentally slower than usual; taking longer to finish things, feeling disorganized, with slower thinking and processing
- Trouble learning new things
- Trouble multitasking
- Fumbling for the right word or phrase, like being unable to find the right words to finish a sentence
- Having trouble following a conversation or initiating one
- Having trouble finding your way around
- Feeling sluggish or tired or not having energy
- Feeling clumsy, as if something's wrong with your motor skills

What causes chemo brain? Despite its name, chemo brain may happen for different reasons. It can be caused by the cancer itself, by chemotherapy treatment, or by secondary medical conditions such as anemia. While it is most commonly connected with chemotherapy, other treatments, such as additional endocrine therapy, radiation, and surgery, may be associated with it, too—not to mention the inflammation that can result from these treatments. In other words, cancer patients can experience chemo brain even though they haven't had chemotherapy.

Anyone can develop cognitive problems before, during, or after receiving treatment. No matter the duration, chemo brain can severely disrupt quality of life and affect performance both at work and at home. Usually, chemo brain is a short-term issue, and cognitive function usually improves after the end of therapy. Most of the time, the foggy sensation fades away six to twelve months after the cancer is successfully treated. However, in some cases, the symptoms may last for months, sometimes years, after the end of treatment. These long-term cognitive difficulties need acknowledging and addressing.

As always, nobody is suggesting that patients decline or avoid treatment. Far from it. I am sharing this information because it's important to know what these procedures involve, from a whole-body and brain perspective. The goal is not to endanger anybody's life by getting them to go off cancer medications, but to draw attention to these largely understudied issues.

Is Chemo Brain a Sign of Dementia?

The fact that estrogen blockers and aromatase inhibitors suppress estrogen function has spurred concerns around a possible risk of dementia. The tricky thing here is that endocrine (hormonal) therapy can be done with or without chemotherapy, and the effects of these two treatments are difficult to tell apart. Nonetheless, several studies have shown that chemotherapy is the major culprit behind the brain fog and memory lapses, whereas endocrine therapy has more variable effects, which depend on several factors, especially the patient's age and type of treatment. For example, tamoxifen—the most common estrogen blocker typically given to women who are not yet in menopause—can have negative effects on memory and speech production. It goes without saying that if a woman is receiving both chemotherapy and tamoxifen, her brain fog may be worse than with either type of treatment by itself. On the other hand, aromatase inhibitors don't seem to have clear negative effects on cognitive performance, at least in postmenopausal women.

Specifically for Alzheimer's disease, although research on this topic is scant, some studies have shown that patients treated with tamoxifen don't have an increased risk of dementia as compared to patients on other treatments. How can this be? While tamoxifen blocks estrogen receptors in breast tissue, it has neutral or positive effects in other parts of the body. It is possible, then, that after a temporary negative impact on cognitive performance, the drug may have mild or no long-term effects overall. As for aromatase inhibitors, there are some differences between steroidal and nonsteroidal formulations. Exemestane, a steroidal aromatase inhibitor, has been linked with a possibly lower risk of dementia than the nonsteroidal drugs anastrozole and letrozole. While more research is sorely needed to confirm these findings, this information can already help support conversations with medical providers about both the cancer and a patient's brain health, as current guidelines permit the choice between different treatment regimens. Personally, I'd also argue for a more integrative approach to cancer care that includes brain specialists besides oncologists and surgeons. Whenever there is a real concern about cognitive impairment or dementia, or when patients continue to struggle with significant cognitive concerns and functional reintegration six to twelve months after the end of treatment, a proper neurological evaluation with brain imaging and neuropsychological testing can make all the difference.

Just as important, I want to be clear that chemo brain and perceived declines in cognitive power do not necessarily constitute cognitive impairment, no matter what words your doctor chooses to use. While it is true that many cancer patients experience a decline in cognitive performance during or after treatment, these changes are hardly ever severe enough to fall in the "impaired" range of cognition—let alone meet an actual diagnosis of impaired cognitive status or dementia. Unfortunately many providers fail to recognize this important distinction and use the term *impairment* to describe any decline in cognitive performance, whether measurable or perceived. We need to be more mindful of our choice of words. Telling patients they are cognitively impaired when they are not can have negative effects on their quality of life, as well as on their stress and anxiety levels, not to mention their self-esteem. In the clearest possible terms, suffering from chemo brain *does not mean one is developing dementia*. As challenging and frightening as these symptoms can be, our powerful brains have the ability to push through and recover. In cases where the recovery seems challenging, seeking guidance from a brain expert can provide valuable support and insights. If you have genuine concerns about dementia, particularly if the symptoms of chemo brain persist or if you have a family history of dementia, I recommend consulting with a neurologist or gerontologist. By conducting targeted assessments, including blood work, cognitive evaluations and specific brain scans, these specialists can provide guidance regarding the best course of action.

Treating Chemo Brain

If you are experiencing chemo brain and the symptoms are causing trouble in your daily life, ask your doctor if you might be helped by a specialist such as a psychologist or psychotherapist, neuropsychologist, speech-language pathologist, occupational therapist, or vocational therapist. These professionals can test you and recommend ways to help you better handle the problems you are experiencing. More generally, things that are proven to help include:

- Cognitive rehabilitation, involving activities to improve brain function, such as learning how the brain works and ways to take in new information and perform new tasks; doing some activities over and over that become harder with time; and using tools to help stay organized, such as planners or diaries.
- Exercise, and more broadly, keeping physically active is good for both your body and your brain, improving your mood, making you feel more alert, and decreasing fatigue.
- Meditation can increase your focus and awareness, while reducing stress.
- Rest and sleep can help your body and brain adjust and heal.
- Avoiding alcohol, caffeine, and other stimulants that might change your mental state and sleeping patterns.
- Asking for help. Tell family members, friends, and your cancer care team about any struggles. Their support and understanding can help you relax and make it easier for you to focus on healing.

I HAD/HAVE BREAST AND/OR OVARIAN CANCER: CAN I TAKE HRT?

While the above practices are well accepted in the medical community, the role of HRT in easing chemo brain and the long-term effects of induced menopause in cancer patients are the subject of fierce debate. Most experts feel that nonhormonal therapies should be the first approach in managing menopausal symptoms in breast and ovarian cancer survivors. We talked about nonhormonal medications in chapter 10 and will go over many lifestyle options in part 4 of this book. When it comes to HRT, according to professional societies, there is a lack of safety data supporting the use of systemic (oral or transdermal) HRT in women who have had breast or ovarian cancer. The risk of breast cancer recurrence with HRT is higher in those with estrogen receptor positive cancer, but patients with estrogen receptor negative breast cancer may also have an increased risk of the cancer regrowing. Nonetheless, HRT may (the North American Menopause Society adds "in exceptional cases") be offered to patients with severe menopausal symptoms if lifestyle modifications and nonhormonal options are not effective. Additionally, hormone therapy "can be considered in premenopausal women who undergo oophorectomy to completely remove the cancer, based on considerations of the many benefits of estrogen therapy for early menopause." As a reminder, for the vast majority of women, low-dose vaginal estradiol and DHEA (a hormone the body can convert into estrogen and testosterone) are safe and effective at treating symptoms such as vaginal dryness and genitourinary symptoms, without noticeable increases in blood estrogen levels.

All this only further highlights the need to engage in comprehensive and individualized discussions with your healthcare team so as to make informed decisions that prioritize both your medical care and symptom management, while also considering your personal risk tolerance. These discussions will enable you to navigate the complexities of treatment options and tailor them to your specific needs. I look forward to the next generation of brain estrogens, or SERMs, becoming available, too. As we discussed in the last chapter, SERMs can be engineered to selectively supply estrogen to the brain while having neutral or even protective effects on reproductive organs. Once this type of therapy is fully tested, there is hope that it will be safe for all women, cancer patients included.

What If I Have a Family History of Breast or Ovarian Cancer?

In 2013, Angelina Jolie disclosed that she had a genetic mutation linked to a strong risk of breast and ovarian cancer. The gene involved is BRCA-1. Its mutations account for about 12 percent of all cases of breast cancers and for another 10 to 15 percent of ovarian cancers. Although she did not have cancer herself, Ms. Jolie decided to take preventative action and have her breasts and ovaries removed. By doing so, she reduced her risk of both cancers back to baseline levels. Ms. Jolie's medical decision hit a nerve with many women around the world. Her story was so impactful that it undoubtedly led to a bevy of women calling their doctor's office for appointments for genetic counseling and breast screening—and questions about what to do next.

If you've been there, you know. If you end up having your ovaries removed, prompting early menopause, would it be safe to take HRT? Would the recommendation of starting HRT as soon as possible after oophorectomy apply to those with genetic mutations, or a family history of breast cancer, or both?

HRT is indeed an option. Several studies indicate that hormone therapy is viable for women who have genetic mutations or a family history of breast cancer, but do not *personally* have the cancer. The same applies to mutation carriers who opt for preventative surgery. So if you or someone you know is in this situation and exploring potential options, it may be helpful to know that HRT is on the table. Nonhormonal and lifestyle modifications should be given equal consideration as they, too, play a significant role in managing menopausal symptoms and supporting brain health. Ultimately, the choice should be based on a comprehensive assessment of individual circumstances and a shared decision-making process between each patient and their healthcare providers.

MOVING BEYOND FEAR, TOGETHER

In my line of work, I am often reminded of how blessed I am to have not only my health but also medical insurance and access to hospitals—not to mention an education that helps me ask the right questions, sort through difficult and often unclear information, and make informed decisions for myself and my family.

I am here today, determined to put my privilege to good use for all women around me. I am powerfully aware that somewhere else in the world, perhaps just in the room next door, there's a woman just like me, with similar abilities and love for her family, who is waiting to find out if she has cancer or needs surgery or she's past treatment. She might be worrying about being able to afford the visit or getting laid off for missing work—or wondering if she'll live long enough to see her kids grow.

Here in the United States, one in every eight women will develop breast cancer in her lifetime. One in every nine will have an oophorectomy, many due to cancer. One in every four will undergo induced menopause.

I stand strong in my determination that women who undergo any of these realities are true warriors. They have a different approach to life, a different look in their eye. They've confronted their own humanity in such a profound way. They've stood up to danger and stigma and fear and all the craziness of the medical establishment, which offers so little support to menopausal women in general and to cancer survivors in particular. Many of you may have already had this dreaded disease and will have wisdom to share with us. On my end, I will do the best I can with my time, my knowledge, and my voice to support and validate all women's stories and experiences and to make sure no voice gets subsumed in the noise of a communal narrative that doesn't reflect any of these realities. To this aim, I launched an entire clinical research program dedicated to women's health, and I'm hoping this book enables more women to become aware of these challenges and learn about possible solutions. Many others will hopefully feel renewed compassion, if not a sense of duty and responsibility toward those who are less fortunate and in need of help.

The ultimate goal, of course, is better solutions and better care for all. So far, we have reviewed the risks and benefits of hormonal therapies for cancer, the dos and don'ts of HRT, and the realistic alternatives provided by nonhormonal medications. Additionally, in part 4, we'll go over several options cancer survivors have to safeguard their mind-body health as they progress through their healing journey. These options do not involve taking hormones or medications—they involve optimizing your lifestyle and environment in ways that are conducive to brain health. For a quick preview, lifestyle and behavioral techniques that are proven to help include dietary management with appropriate supplements and specific exercise regimens, as well as cognitive behavioral therapy, hypnosis, and relaxation techniques. Remember, there is power in your everyday choices. This is an important concept and one I hope you, too, will take to heart.

12

Gender-Affirming Therapy

SEX AND GENDER

In previous chapters, we have used the term *women* to discuss individuals born with two X chromosomes and reproductive characteristics such as breasts and ovaries, commonly known as cisgender women. This combination has long been the biological definition of the female sex. While the binary notion of female or male, XX or XY, is deeply ingrained in our society, the understanding of gender has evolved over time. In medical science, we acknowledge that possessing a female reproductive system does not dictate one's gender identity. Some individuals do not identify with the sex they were assigned at birth, rather expressing gender on a spectrum, leading to the expansion of the LGBTQ community into the LGBTQIA+ community (lesbian, gay, bisexual, transgender, queer or questioning, intersex, asexual) in recent decades.

Transgender individuals, who represent around 0.5 percent of the U.S. population, and intersex individuals, who account for approximately 2 percent, often face significant challenges in accessing appropriate healthcare. Many medical providers lack training in transgender care in particular, leaving up to half of all transgender individuals in the position of having to inform their providers about their specific needs. Now add hormones to the mix, and the picture becomes even more complex. Accessible providers who specialize in gender-affirming therapies, which may include hormonal and surgical treatments, generally do so with regard to the patient's *body*. Few are prepared to manage their patients' cognitive and mental well-being, too.

In our exploration of hormones' effects on brain health, we will now consider the experiences of transgender individuals who undergo hormonal transitions during their gender-affirming therapy. This chapter discusses transgender men in particular, who were assigned the female sex at birth but who have transitioned to a male or masculine gender and may unknowingly be experiencing brain changes related to both the treatment and to hormonal changes due to, or not unlike, menopause. These brain-body changes are much less researched and understood than hormonal transitions occurring in cisgender women, making reliable information on the topic especially challenging to find. We will also talk about transgender women, who were assigned the male sex at birth and have transitioned to a female or feminine gender, as they, too, may encounter similar challenges.

While I am not a psychologist or sociologist and must defer to other professionals regarding the emotional and social aspects of gender transition, I am committed to understanding how the hormonal changes that may occur can impact an individual's health and cognitive well-being. Beyond my desire to make sure that this book is inclusive, another reason to discuss how gender-affirming therapies impact the brain is that the treatment of choice for transgender men often involves the use of testosterone paired with estrogen-suppressing medications, which may provoke either menopause itself or some of its symptoms. A better understanding of the effect of these treatments will not only support further progress in transgender care but also contribute to a more comprehensive understanding of the diverse experiences of all people undergoing this hormonal milestone.

GENDER IDENTITY: A PRIMER

Some may feel nonplussed about what transgender identity is and isn't. Others may confuse it with homosexuality. Here's a good place to start: Sexuality is about to whom you're attracted. Gender identity is about who you feel you *are* gender-wise. One's gender identity can be separate from one's sexual preference.

Let's go a little deeper. Cisgender women identify with the sex assigned to them at birth. They were born with a reproductive system assigned female and are at ease with their given genitalia and associated gender identity. Ditto for cisgender men who were born with genitalia assigned male and associate with that gender identity. Transgender individuals, on the other hand, identify with the gender opposite their assigned sex. In medical textbooks, the incongruence between one's sense of gender and one's sex assigned at birth or social presentation is called *gender dysphoria*. Gender dysphoria is a broader concept than just physical attributes. Trans people can have body dysphoria and/or social dysphoria. One or the other may present more strongly. Generally, the discomfort of being in a body that does not feel like your own or that doesn't match your identity can cause considerable psychological suffering, increasing the risk of stress, anxiety, and depression in turn.

Gender-Affirming Therapy

People who are transgender may pursue multiple domains of gender affirmation, including social affirmation (e.g., changing one's name and pronouns), legal affirmation (e.g., changing gender markers on one's government-issued documents), medical affirmation (e.g., pubertal suppression or gender-affirming hormones), and/or surgical affirmation (e.g., vaginoplasty, facial surgery, breast augmentation, masculine chest reconstruction, etc.). Of note, not all people who are transgender will desire all domains of gender affirmation, as these are highly personal and individual decisions.

Herein, I'll focus on medical gender-affirming therapy (GAT), or cross-sex therapy, which transgender and gender nonbinary individuals are increasingly using to intercept their transition to puberty, or to match their gender identity post-puberty. Medical GAT therefore includes a transition, with hormones or surgery in some cases. GAT is generally used to reduce the bodily characteristics of a person's natal sex while inducing those of the gender they identify with. Hormonal treatment is the more commonly used route. Fewer transgender people elect to have surgery, whether because of social, medical, or financial considerations, or just personal preference. These complementary procedures and assistance are associated with improved quality of life and mental health for many transgender individuals.

There are two main types of GAT, depending on which gender one is transitioning to:

▶ MASCULINIZING HORMONE THERAPY (OR TRANSMASCULINE, FEMALE-TO-MALE HORMONE THERAPY)

Masculinizing hormone therapy is the GAT predominantly used by transgender men as well as other transmasculine and intersex individuals. The purpose is to change the secondary sexual characteristics from feminine or androgynous to masculine, transforming the body into one more congruent with a male gender identity. Masculinizing therapy typically prompts voice deepening and the development of a masculine pattern of hair, fat, and muscle distribution. If started before puberty, GAT can prevent some breast and vulva development. If started after puberty, GAT cannot undo breast and vulva development, which may be addressed by surgery and other treatments.

The mainstay of masculinizing therapy is testosterone. Several formulations are available, including intramuscular injections, transdermal patches, gels, pellets, and pills. Anti-estrogen therapies are also used to reduce the body's production of estrogen and progesterone. Some of these medicines are called gonadotropin-releasing hormone (GnRH) antagonists. The term *antagonists* refers to the fact that these drugs work against the release of LH and FSH hormones. This in turn stops the production of estrogen and progesterone in the ovaries. Some estrogen blockers and aromatase inhibitors, like the drugs used for cancer treatment discussed in the last chapter, can also be used. Additionally, some transgender men choose surgeries to remove the breasts, uterus, and/or ovaries, and may elect to undergo reconstructive surgeries afterward. These changes additionally alter the hormonal milieu of transgender men.

In terms of timeline, increased body hair growth, scalp hair loss, and an increase in muscle mass and strength usually occur within a year of starting masculinizing therapy. The menstrual cycle stops after just two to six months of treatment. The one thing that this treatment doesn't necessarily stop is ovulation. This exception means that transgender men can become pregnant (unless contraception is used) and that they will go through menopause when the time comes. As we find new ways to honor the fluidity of gender, we bump into the fact that our physiological sex may not be as flexible as our gender identity. So to be clear, if a person is born with ovaries and has had a menstrual cycle at some point in their lives, they will inevitably go through menopause.

So here we are looking at a *double* transition—one for gender affirmation and the other for menopause. These transitions can intertwine, potentially complicating each other. For transgender men, menopause can happen spontaneously, over time, or as a result of surgery. Transgender men who undergo an oophorectomy (the surgical removal of the ovaries, possibly along with the uterus) will develop menopause soon after surgery, incurring the same risks as a cisgender woman undergoing induced menopause. As discussed throughout the book, oophorectomies before menopause may increase a person's risk of developing heart disease and osteoporosis, as well as anxiety, depression, and even cognitive impairment in older age. Unfortunately, transgender men are seldom offered adequate preparation for what menopause involves, whether spontaneous or induced. It is my hope this book will help provide clarity on what to expect and how to mitigate possible symptoms and side effects.

▶ **FEMINIZING HORMONE THERAPY (TRANSFEMININE OR MALE-TO-FEMALE HORMONE THERAPY)**

Feminizing hormone therapy is the GAT predominantly used by transgender women as well as other transfeminine and intersex people. In this case, GAT is used to feminize their bodies. Treatment typically involves oral, transdermal, or injectable estrogen preparations, often in conjunction with GnRH analogs. These GnRH drugs stimulate estrogen and progesterone production (as opposed to the GnRH antagonists mentioned above). Anti-androgen medicines can also be used, in this case to suppress testosterone.

Does GAT Change the Brain?

Now that we've reviewed the main types of GAT, let's return to my wheelhouse: brain health. Do masculinizing and feminizing treatments have any notable effects on the brain?

It is important to note that introducing external hormones while dramatically reducing the body's own hormonal production impacts the entire body, the brain included. While the effects of hormones on appearance and sexual characteristics are self-evident, we've yet to compile adequate clinical research on how GAT impacts the brain. Research on transgender individuals is still in its infancy, and the majority of whatever few studies have been carried out focus on transgender women. There are hardly any brain studies of transgender men, highlighting, once again, the healthcare stigma and marginalization discussed throughout this book. Another issue is that most studies so far have limited themselves to young transgender individuals in their early twenties and thirties, if not younger. Nonetheless, let's take a look at what we have to work with so far.

As discussed at the beginning of this book, research on cisgender individuals has shown that men's and women's brains have some differences. Those most often cited are that men's brains tend to be bigger overall and women's brains tend to be more interconnected. These facts are interesting to ponder, as we review the impact of GAT on the brain.

Some studies have used MRI scans to look at the brain before and after GAT treatment in transgender individuals, mostly transgender women. The scans allowed the researchers to take a peek at the brain's gray matter to monitor if it was thicker or thinner after feminizing GAT, simultaneously measuring any changes in connectivity between brain regions near and far. The results are intriguing. After six months to a year of treatment with anti-testosterone medicines, some specific brain regions of transgender women had indeed grown smaller, whereas their connectivity had increased. In other words, GAT prompted the brains of transgender women to exhibit some of the structural characteristics of a cisgender female brain, being typically smaller and more interconnected relative to those of cisgender men. While there are fewer studies of this transition, this mirror crossover is seen in transgender men, too. In this case, treatment with testosterone and anti-estrogen medicines had the exact opposite effect on the brain, increasing its volume overall, as well as in several regions typically larger in cisgender men. Overall, GAT appears to align a person's brain with those characteristics comparable to the gender with which the person identifies, at least to some degree. These results also suggest that GAT changes the brain as surely as it does the body, perhaps in ways that may help relieve the feeling of incongruence between one's body and gender identity. However, what may come as a surprise is that these changes may simultaneously impact a person's mood, energy levels, sleep patterns, cognitive performance, and even long-term health, as discussed below.

How Do These Changes Impact One's Health?

From a clinical perspective, besides the desired changes in bodily appearance, GAT has some additional pros and cons. For example, transgender men receiving testosterone therapy tend to report increased energy, focus, appetite, and libido, along with a decreased need for sleep. That's the good news. The not-so-good news is that treatment may trigger hot flashes, brain fog, depressive episodes, and other brain symptoms of menopause. These changes may be more severe when the ovaries are removed, which can occur as early as puberty if that's when the surgery occurs. Masculinizing GAT can also cause vaginal atrophy and dryness. In this case, topical estrogen creams and lubricants can help (see chapter 9). In the long term, this type of treatment may increase the risk of osteoporosis and polycystic ovary syndrome (PCOS), which, if left untreated, has been linked to decreased fertility and a possible increased risk of endometrial cancer. These risks are important to acknowledge and address, as are those related to undergoing an oophorectomy before the natural age of menopause.

Transgender women may experience somewhat opposite changes after anti-testosterone and/or estrogen therapy, such as reduced libido and alterations in mood, sleep, and temperature sensitivity. This is also not too different from menopause brain. According to some studies looking at long-term effects, transgender women on GAT may have a higher risk of heart disease and breast cancer than cisgender men.

GAT's Effects on Cognitive Performance

Given all that we've come to understand about the effects of hormonal changes on brain health, one can't help but wonder if GAT could also impact cognitive functioning. For the time being, we need more information, as research on the long-term risks and benefits of GAT is still minimal, and the few existing studies on the topic are also limited to young transgender individuals, mostly transgender women. Nonetheless, the most extensive study so far, combining data from several hundred young adult transgender men and women, indicates no clear negative effects in the short term. Rather, transgender men on testosterone therapy showed somewhat enhanced visuospatial performance, while transgender women on estrogen therapy exhibited a slight improvement in verbal memory. If you recall from previous chapters, while the jury's still out as to whether cognitive differences can be reliably found between the genders, these results align with those cognitive strengths comparable to the gender with which the person identifies (cisgender women tend to have better verbal memory than cisgender men, while cisgender men may have better visuospatial abilities than cisgender women).

That said, it is baffling that virtually nothing is known about GAT effects among transgender people over thirty, transgender men in particular. We have yet to collect enough reliable information on how GAT and menopause combined could impact cognitive and mental health in groups of people, let alone for each individual. This duo is a noteworthy one to examine, especially given the higher rates of anxiety and depression experienced by many transgender individuals already before menopause. While we develop the studies necessary to guide and protect transgender people through their transitions with care and know-how, for now we await additional data to assess GAT's fuller impact on cognition.

This waiting game makes preventative care all the more essential. As we wait for the data to roll in, my advice is the same for transgender individuals as it is for everybody else. As we've come to understand just how critical hormones are to a myriad of brain functions and how menopause may impact those brain functions, we must take excellent care as we pioneer the process. My best advice is to treat your brain as your best friend and show it your utmost respect, at all ages and stages of life. This book is here to ensure that you are prioritizing your brain and mental health using scientifically validated techniques that are proven to work. As our culture and medical field integrate the latest findings from the front lines, it's up to us to fortify our brain's well-being using the tools discussed in these pages.

PART 4

LIFESTYLE AND INTEGRATIVE HEALTH

13

Exercise

THE POWER OF LIFESTYLE

So far we've discussed prescription medicines that can help alleviate the symptoms of menopause and support you through this journey. However, many women prefer to rely on natural remedies, diet, and exercise instead. Fortunately, this is perfectly feasible, and a wide array of lifestyle changes and self-care practices are available. Importantly, these techniques are just as valuable if HRT or other medications are part of your plan.

When it comes to lifestyle, menopause is a great moment to select new healthy habits and to keep consistent with positive current ones. In this spirit, I want you to think of your brain as a muscle. You can incorporate behaviors that strengthen the brain, just as you train your muscles. You can exercise it, feed it properly, take care of it properly—and when you do, your brain will perform much better for you, at any age. Things like eating a nutritious diet, avoiding toxins, and keeping stress under control can really make a difference, as do exercise, sleep, and a mindset fueled with facts, not fiction. Your body and brain will take care of you if you take care of them.

Harnessing this prescribed lifestyle's power can influence how your brain *responds* to menopause, making you feel better, lighter, and brighter on your way. If you are having a hard time during the period leading up to menopause, it's helpful to remember that you have agency over your lifestyle, environment, and beliefs. These factors can play a significant role in shaping your experience of menopause. Just as hormonal changes can affect your sleep, focus, and body composition, your daily habits can also influence your hormone levels and the intensity of their effects on your body.

I want to make clear that I am not here to download a to-do list to "overcome" or "beat" menopause. Remember, menopause is not an enemy. Above all, I am not interested in selling you on a program that will make your brain impervious to menopause or magically propel you beyond it. That's just science fiction. The vetted lifestyle choices discussed ahead are based on tried-and-true research. Tangible benefits are feasible with time, consistency, and persistence. Let's go!

EXERCISE FOR A HEALTHY MENOPAUSE

It'll probably come as no surprise that most of us aren't on the move nearly as much as would be optimal, not even close! According to the U.S. Centers for Disease Control and Prevention (CDC), less than 40 percent of adults engage in even two and a half hours of physical activity per week. And guess what—women in their forties and older are by far the highest demographic to exercise inconsistently. Many don't exercise at all. This drop-off in physical activity comes at a cost and couldn't come at a worse time.

There's no shortage of good reasons to be physically active. If you're approaching menopause, there are even more. Physical activity can trigger positive hormonal changes that directly reduce the number and severity of hot flashes, improve mood, and enhance sleep. It supports cognitive strength, too, while boosting your stamina and enhancing your quality of life. This news alone should get you on your feet. But there's more. Medical conditions that often make menopause worse or like to pop up simultaneously with it, like metabolic issues and insulin resistance, can be reduced or even *reversed* by exercising. Regular physical activity can help lower the risk of a seemingly endless list of chronic diseases, including heart disease, stroke, high blood pressure, type 2 diabetes, osteoporosis, obesity, colon cancer, breast cancer, anxiety, depression, and even dementia! If there was a pill for that, we'd all be taking it. What if we picked a combo of exercises we liked instead?

Think about it like this: When it comes to our bodies, everything is connected, and there is an undeniable domino effect at work. Exercise can stabilize your blood sugar levels, giving you more energy, which in and of itself will likely put you in a better mood. More vitality and a better outlook might prompt you to keep exercising over time, aiding in weight management. Weight management is a great way to keep hot flashes at bay while boosting your confidence. A drop in the number of hot flashes improves your sleep quality, which can help you manage stress. And so forth. Over time, these reciprocal relationships create a positive flow inside our bodies and in our lives, turning a vicious cycle into a victorious one. Exercise can be a way to take over the reins in menopause, enjoying a new, steady gallop where we'd once felt at the mercy of a wild horse.

There are no two ways about it. Maintaining a consistent exercise regimen is a realistic goal for those who wish to have a healthier, smoother menopause while setting themselves up for lifelong wellness. The bonanza of bonuses exercise brings to the table is evident on multiple fronts, a few of which I'm highlighting for you in the following text.

Healthy Weight and Metabolism

Around menopause, many women witness an increase in body fat they just can't explain. It's bad enough that your sleep is disrupted by hot flashes that rival the fires of Mount Vesuvius, and that as a result your stress levels are off the charts, but now your formerly comfy jeans have turned on you, too. It's understandable to feel frustrated and confused. But don't scratch your head—we've caught the culprit.

It's a combo attack. When aging, menopause, and a decrease in physical activity gang up on you, it can lead to a decline in your metabolic rate and lean muscle. Midlife women tend to gain an average of 4 to 5 pounds over just a few years. Waist size also increases by about 2.2 centimeters (about 1 inch). However, contrary to popular belief, while aging *may* cause weight gain, menopause itself does not. It can, however, increase your belly fat. How so? Fluctuating levels of estrogen can trigger fat storage in the body, and the belly is the storage shed. However inconvenient this may seem, there is a method to this madness. As ovarian production of estradiol slows down, our body relies on belly fat tissue to produce estrone, estrogen's backup. We actually need that belly fat to ensure that some estrogen production continues as we age. However, while having enough body fat can help maintain our hormonal health, too much can cause other problems, as we know. This shift can result in an apple body shape, usually accompanied by a buildup of visceral fat—a stealth fat that collects around internal organs, increasing the risk of heart disease and metabolic disorders. It's also true that the drop in estrogen can result in fatigue, achy joints, and reduced stamina, making hitting the couch look a lot more inviting than hopping off it.

For some good news, the possible increases in weight and waistline are *temporary* for most women, slowing a few years postmenopause. Most important, none of this is inevitable. In fact, one of the many ways exercise benefits you is by stoking your metabolism and stabilizing your weight. This assist is particularly helpful as several studies show that perimenopausal and postmenopausal women who engage in regular physical activity can greatly improve their body composition, achieving a lower body mass index (BMI), less belly fat, and a higher metabolism, which allows them to burn calories more easily *no matter their age.*

Reduced Risk of Heart Disease and Diabetes

Heart disease remains the number one cause of death in women over fifty. This may be related to the loss of estrogen's beneficial effects on our vascular system, combined with a midlife increase in "bad" LDL (low density lipoprotein) cholesterol. The additional accumulation of abdominal fat during menopause can increase the risk of insulin resistance and type 2 diabetes (risk factors for heart disease, in turn).

But get this: Exercise can lessen or even reverse these risks. As little as twelve weeks of training can improve weight, decrease waist circumference, and lower triglycerides and total cholesterol in menopausal women. At the same time, it promotes healthy blood pressure at all ages. Not for nothing, women under sixty who maintain a regular exercise routine have a much lower risk of heart disease in their seventies and eighties. The bottom line: Physical activity promotes heart health, and what's good for the heart is good for the brain—not to mention the rest of you!

Reduced Hot Flashes

Exercise's power to minimize and potentially prevent menopause-related symptoms is making headlines worldwide. Well-established professional societies such as the North American Menopause Society and the UK's Royal College of Obstetricians and Gynaecologists recommend regular exercise as a valuable intervention for keeping hot flashes at bay. That's because exercise improves the body's ability to regulate its temperature, making us less likely to slam and jam our perspiration button. As mentioned earlier, exercise also helps regulate body and fat mass. This one-two punch can dramatically decrease the number and severity of hot flashes! In clinical trials, women who started out with excess body fat and lost weight by exercising during the course of the study reported meaningful reductions in, and sometimes complete elimination of, hot flashes in as little as one year.

Additionally, if hot flashes do occur, the amount of sweating and discomfort is significantly reduced in women who exercise regularly. In a study of 3,500 Latin American women, those who engaged in regular moderate-intensity exercise were 28 percent less likely to have severe hot flashes than those who exercised less. In a sample of over 400 Australian women, those exercising daily experienced 49 percent fewer hot flashes than those who were sedentary. This is quite impressive if you consider that taking HRT can reduce hot flashes by about 75 percent. The best news yet is that these benefits can be recouped starting right now, even without a history of regular exercise. According to several studies, sedentary women who take up a fitness routine for the first time in their lives and stick with it can experience a marked reduction in hot flashes in as little as three months' time.

Better Sleep

The truth is, physically active women sleep better. Higher levels of sedentary time are consistently associated with poorer sleep, if not full-blown insomnia—all major concerns among women going through menopause. On the other hand, physically active perimenopausal and postmenopausal women awaken less during the night, have an improved quality of sleep, and suffer less from insomnia.

Better Mood and a Sense of Well-Being

When we exercise, *endorphins*, our body's natural painkillers, flow freely, automatically lifting our spirits. Serotonin releases, relaxing and "happifying" us. This antidepressant effect is linked to a drop in stress hormones, and everyone could use some of that. The result: Midlife women with greater physical activity consistently report a better quality of life, a heightened sense of psychological well-being, and reduced symptoms of depression and anxiety—both before and after menopause. In a combined analysis of eleven clinical trials totaling almost 2,000 midlife women, regular exercise significantly reduced depressive symptoms, as well as stress and related insomnia, after just twelve weeks. Both moderate and low-intensity exercise regimens worked like a charm. Since not everyone is into (or capable of) high-intensity workouts, this is good news indeed.

Better Memory and a Lower Risk of Dementia

Exercise is not only muscle-building, stress-busting, and endorphin-releasing—it is also memory-enhancing. For example, in a study of thousands of elderly people, those who engaged in regular physical activity had a 35 percent lower risk of developing dementia than those who were sedentary. You should note that many of these activities were not in gyms but were done in street clothes, like walking, biking, climbing stairs, and doing household chores.

For our purposes, a recent study followed about 200 midlife women for as long as forty-four years. The results show that those with the highest level of cardiovascular fitness in midlife had a whopping 30 percent lower risk of developing dementia as they got older compared to those who remained sedentary. As a dementia specialist, I can assure you that a 30 percent reduction in the rates of dementia is nothing short of extraordinary—so far, no drug has achieved such an effect. Sure enough, our brain-imaging studies also demonstrate that physically active midlife women exhibit more vigorous brain activity, less brain shrinkage, and fewer Alzheimer's plaques as compared to their sedentary counterparts. These fantastic results contribute to maintaining a clear head and long-lasting memories.

Stronger Bones and Fewer Injuries

One of exercise's most sought-after benefits is the miracle it works on bone density. When we strengthen our muscles, we strengthen our bones. Physical activity effectively slows bone loss after menopause, lowering the risk of fractures and osteoporosis. Reducing the likelihood of falls and injuries improves our mobility and reduces our pain potential, during menopause and beyond.

Increased Longevity

The following is not hyperbole: Staying active can actually save your life. It is not my intention to freak you out with the statistics below, but let's not mince words—the more time you spend sitting and lying down with little to no exercise, the higher your risk of, well, dying.

To give you some examples, in the Women's Health Initiative, among over 92,000 postmenopausal women ages fifty to seventy-nine, those who reported the lowest amounts of sedentary time showed a significantly reduced risk of mortality compared to their physically inactive counterparts. Specifically, those who spent more than five hours per day being physically active were 27 percent less likely to die of heart disease and 21 percent less likely to die of cancer than those who spent eight hours or more per day in sedentary mode. (Ah, no, that doesn't include time spent sleeping.) More striking evidence comes from the Nurses' Health Study, which revealed similar findings among younger women, ages thirty-four to fifty-nine. When these women reached their seventies and eighties, those who had been physically active had a 77 percent lower risk of respiratory death, a 31 percent lower risk of dying from heart disease, and a 13 percent lower risk of dying from cancer than those who were mostly sedentary. Well then, time to get moving.

WHAT KIND OF EXERCISE IS BEST?

Everyone struggles to find enough me time. Is there some way we can exercise *smarter* rather than *harder*? Are there certain kinds of exercise that favor women of menopausal age? How about older women? The top questions about training are how hard, how often, how long, and what type of exercise can really make the cut.

How Often

- *Before menopause.* Here the target is four to five 45-to-60-minute sessions a week. Research shows this formula is particularly effective at supporting hormonal health and even fertility. Remember, the longer you're fertile, the later you go through menopause.
- *For traversing menopause through age sixty-five or so.* During this period we tailor the recipe to three to five days a week, at 30 to 60 minutes a clip, and adjust the duration and intensity of the workout based on age, severity of symptoms, and overall health and fitness level. Obviously, if you can do more, do more.
- *After age seventy.* Daily sessions of at least 15 minutes each are a good rule of thumb, though many women can (and will) do more than this.

How Hard

There's a recurrent myth that the older you get, the harder you have to exercise to see results. Rigorous research on this topic shows precisely the opposite. Especially for postmenopausal women, moderate-intensity exercise serves you *better* than intense bursts of effort. Remember, we're not talking about bodybuilding here; we are targeting your overall health.

In midlife, the relationship between exercise intensity and health looks like an upside-down U. As shown in figure 9, a low-intensity exercise yields some health gains, but moderate-intensity is where the action is, providing the maximum return. Increasing your workouts to a high-intensity range doesn't seem to improve the benefits; perhaps surprisingly, it shows diminishing returns. Regular moderate-intensity exercise has been linked to the lowest risk of heart disease, stroke, diabetes, and cancer in women, starting around midlife. As another incentive, it's also associated with better sleep.

Figure 9. Exercise intensity and health gains in midlife women

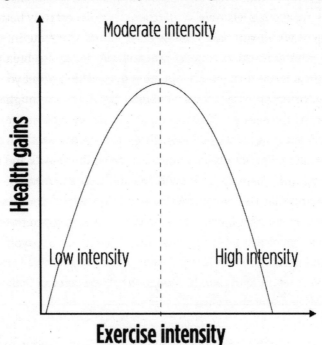

With all the buzz around boot camps, boxing, stationary biking (spinning), and high-intensity interval training, you might wonder why moderate-intensity exercise is so effective. First, it's important to point out that none of the above programs are developed with female physiology in mind, let alone any awareness of menopause. They target trends based on a very specific demographic and then sell the program as good for *everybody*. The truth is, they're not good for everybody. And guess what? Scientists have found that high-intensity training clearly benefits *men*, whereas cardio and resistance training at a moderate intensity work better *for women*. This difference may be because high-intensity exercise increases the stress hormone cortisol—which most women already have plenty of. High-intensity workouts also require more sleep and rest to recover from—an elusive commodity in a woman's world.

Let's clarify what constitutes moderate-intensity exercise. We are not talking about a leisurely stroll (though that's certainly better than nothing, if it's all you have time or energy for). Moderate intensity is any exercise that ups your heart rate and enables you to break a light sweat. To achieve this, you should move fast enough to get your blood flowing, bringing roses to your cheeks. Although you might have a little breathiness when talking, you shouldn't struggle to catch your breath. Singing out loud, however, should be a challenge.

To be clear, I'm not saying ditch your bigger dumbbells and to heck with push-ups. There are plenty who can do all of that and then some. I am saying that the sweet spot for our purposes is exercising more often at a moderate intensity. This rhythm ensures you exercise *consistently* enough at just a high-*enough* intensity to get the payoff you deserve and need.

What Type

For maximum benefit, experts recommend focusing on three types of exercise: aerobic, strengthening, and flexibility and balance.

▶ AEROBIC EXERCISE

If you want more bang for your buck, start with aerobic exercise. This type of exercise has long been praised as most effective for everything under the sun. It raises your heart rate, enhances your blood flow and circulation, and pumps oxygen and nutrients throughout your body. This in turn protects your heart against plaque while clearing your head and sharpening your mind. As if this weren't enough, aerobic exercise is the best regimen to foil hot flashes, too.

But again, you don't need to sign up for CrossFit or start prepping for a marathon to reap its benefits. Walking, hiking, or an elliptical machine all do the trick. Multiple clinical trials report that even an activity as simple as brisk walking can significantly improve your health in as little as three months. *Brisk* means walking in a hurry, like you're late for an appointment. In multiple studies, brisk walking for

30 minutes three times a week was effective at reducing insomnia, irritability, and fatigue in midlife women. It also improved weight and waist circumference and lowered triglycerides and total cholesterol. Plus, walking slows down brain shrinkage, effectively protecting us against brain fog and memory decline. In practical terms, walking 6,000 or more steps per day is associated with a decreased risk of heart disease and diabetes in women ages forty and over. Augmenting that target toward 9,000 to 10,000 steps may lower your risk of dementia, too.

Other examples of properly paced exercise are bike riding at 7 to 10 miles per hour, hopping on the elliptical machine at a steady stride, jumping rope, swimming, exercising in the water, playing tennis, attending group fitness classes, dancing, or stair climbing. Remember that you can combine these things into your own quirky customized routine. Any exercise that keeps you on your feet also helps preserve bone mass and prevent osteoporosis.

For those who don't have the extra time or resources to hit the gym or take long walks, let's remember the accumulated effect of everyday activities like gardening, cleaning the house, and running chores, not to mention running after your kids or grandkids. These activities may not achieve the same effects as more intense exercise, but sources say that engaging in one hour a day of low-intensity physical activities has a favorable effect on menopause symptoms and overall quality of life.

▶ STRENGTHENING

The latest evidence points to the power of pairing up moderate-intensity aerobic exercise with weight-bearing exercises for maximum benefits for women. While aerobic exercise targets metabolic health and reduces hot flashes, these strengthening exercises are particularly effective at reducing anxiety and brightening your mood.

Training with free weights, weight machines, or resistance bands can help add muscle mass to your body, thereby stimulating bone-building and boosting metabolism. Body-weight exercises like push-ups and pull-ups, as well as knee raises, planks, lunges, and squats, also build muscle, support bone health, and improve your core strength and balance. Choose whatever weight or resistance level is just heavy enough to feel the burn when doing 15 reps. Gradually increase the weight or resistance level as you get stronger.

▶ FLEXIBILITY AND BALANCE EXERCISES

These are plentiful and include things like yoga, mat Pilates, tai chi, and stretching. All can improve your coordination, keep you steady on your feet, and ward off falls and arthritis down the line. Yoga and Pilates also incorporate specialized breathwork into the exercises, promoting relaxation and hormonal balance as they tone your core. Studies show that this kind of workout, in particular, can release stress and support quality sleep.

We'll talk more about mind-body techniques in chapter 16, but just to reinforce the importance of balance and flexibility, it's time for a spookily telling test. Can you balance on one leg for 10 seconds or longer?

It turns out that poor balance is linked to frailty in older age, and is also a prime indicator of declining health. Women under seventy years of age are pretty much expected to pass this test without blinking an eye. If that's you, great—now make it a whole minute. If you are older than seventy and complete the task easily, congratulations, you are in better shape than many of your peers. If instead you cannot balance on one foot for 10 seconds, regardless of your age, you may be in jeopardy of nearly double the likelihood of a rapid health decline in the next decade or so. If this isn't motivation to sign up for that yoga class, I don't know what is!

STAY MOTIVATED

Most studies, including many clinical trials, indicate that you should start harvesting the fruits of your labor in as little as twelve weeks when you follow the above guidelines. However, even though most people are aware that exercise is well worth doing, many resist. The most common obstacles are money, time, and motivation.

There's a general misconception that to exercise regularly, one must drop a large chunk of change to join a gym or invest in expensive fitness equipment. But seriously, there's no need. Walking, hiking, running, or riding a bicycle if you have one are free and fun ways to exercise. Smaller pieces of equipment such as an exercise ball, dumbbells, or resistance bands can be used for a variety of exercises and are super-efficient (*and* inexpensive). There are also workout routines that don't require a single piece of equipment, many of which you can find for free online and on YouTube.

Lack of time is a tricky one to solve. Just the same, it might be the most common reason women do not exercise. Our schedules are stuffed with work, family, children, and various other responsibilities, or all of the above, so exercise is tough to fit in. While this is a legitimate challenge, we need to keep our eyes on the prize: more energy, better sleep, better mood, clearer heads, less stress, fewer flashes—and the list goes on. So the question is not whether it's doable but how to make it happen. Whether it's a matter of prioritizing it or finding sneaky ways to slip movement into your daily routine, here are some tips that may help:

- Schedule a time each day for exercise. Write it on your calendar and stick to it as best you can.
- Break it up. If you don't have a 60-minute window to exercise, you might find three 20-minute segments in which you can.
- If you don't have more than 20 minutes, then work out for 20 minutes. Never underestimate the power of a quick workout! There is still an enormous difference in overall health compared to doing nothing at all.
- If you are seriously strapped for time, plank. Get yourself in plank position and hold it for as long as possible. Ten minutes in plank pose may be as challenging as an hour of squats.
- If you worry about what to do with your family while you exercise, find a way to exercise together. Take a family walk, play ball in a park or backyard, go for a bike ride, skip rope, or invest in a small trampoline that you can keep inside. When

my daughter was little, I'd do my yoga routine while she climbed me like a jungle gym. She became my favorite free weight, and I was as popular as going to the playground!

- Look for free classes online. If you have the resources, you might consider finding a personal trainer who will help you develop a routine customized to you and your schedule. Many offer Zoom or Skype sessions, cutting out the commute and making it all the more convenient.

- Track your progress to increase your motivation and staying power. As helpful as various gadgets can be, you don't need an Oura ring or an Apple Watch. There are unlimited ways to keep tabs on your physical activity. Just write down how often and how much you've exercised, what you did, how you felt. If you can get a simple step tracker, that can also help you stay on target.

Finally, persistence is paramount. So many people try a form of exercise that's not a fit and find themselves quitting before they even start. This can happen to the best of us, whether we don't see changes in our bodies fast enough or perhaps get discouraged by unattainable goals. Here's what I think: Forget about the celebrities who look twenty-five when they're in their fifties, especially those setting impossible standards. Remember that they employ entire teams of personal trainers, stylists, surgeons, and chefs to get them camera-ready. Define what fitness and health mean for you instead.

It's also worth considering that some people just don't like to exercise. If this is you, I can't stress enough how important it is to find ways to keep your body moving that you actually enjoy and find sustainable. Some people like the competitive aspect of exercise (sports), some like the social aspect (classes), some love the solitary quality (solo walks), and some enjoy having fun (dancing). Perhaps a daily trip to the gym is not for you. You may enjoy walking or biking outdoors more or doing yoga in the park. Or maybe you do love going to the gym but feel weird going it alone. Then join a class or group, or team up with a workout buddy. On the other hand, if going solo is your thing, go for a walk (shooting for those 6,000 or more steps) or crank up some music and dance like no one is watching. Whatever the case, where there's a will, there's a way. Decide what you value regarding your health goals and be the boss of your wellness. Set realistic, achievable goals for yourself, and approach these goals with self-love instead of self-criticism. Get creative, and you do you.

14

Diet and Nutrition

FOOD FOR THOUGHT

In our society, we focus more on dieting to whittle our waistlines than to *nourish* ourselves. We definitely have this backward! Being selective about what we put in our mouths is central to our health and well-being at any stage of life, and it's just as important when it comes to the health of our brains.

Neuro-nutrition, or nutrition for the brain, is a big part of my world. As a brain scientist, I am acutely aware of the importance of food for brain health. This is for three main reasons. First, our brains rely on specific nutrients to function properly. Second, our brain cells are, in very large part, made of the foods we eat. Meal after meal, day after day, those foods—and more specifically, the nutrients they contain—become the very fabric of our brains. Last, our brain cells are built in a unique way compared to the cells that make up our other organs. Unlike the rest of the body, where cells are constantly rebuilt and re-placed, most of our brain neurons are *irreplaceable*. They are born with us and stick with us for most of our lives. With this in mind, the next time you are torn between eating a meal of fresh whole foods or a greasy fast-food cheeseburger, you may want to pause and decide with which you want to fill your head.

When it comes to women's health, not only does smart nutrition have a proven impact on our body composition and energy levels, but it can also be a powerful ally against aging, disease, and—you guessed it—menopause. The key here is to eat *smart* by focusing on filling your plate with nutrient-dense foods, which are particularly rich in nutrients that work in your favor, such as vitamins, minerals, fiber, complex carbohydrates, lean protein, and healthy fats. Besides being nutritious and delicious, smart foods can reduce inflammation and bolster your resilience against stress; they can brighten your mood and clear your head. They can help you sleep better, feel better, and perform better. On top of that, there is evidence that select foods have a positive impact on hormonal health, easing a woman's monthly cycles, and both delaying the onset of menopause and reducing the frequency and severity of its bothersome symptoms. The reverse, however, is also true. A poor diet can indeed make symptoms worse, hasten the onset of menopause, and make you feel cranky, tired, depleted, and brain fogged. When you're going through perimenopause in particular, you may begin to notice that certain foods trigger certain symptoms. For example, foods that spike blood sugar levels can suddenly zap your energy and leave you more irritable than ever. Drinking alcohol can exaggerate, extend, or multiply hot flashes. Refined, processed, and preservative-heavy foods are expert at taking down your mood and focus, killing two precious birds with one stone.

It is important, then, to learn which foods and nutrients are supportive of our brain health in general—and our brain health in menopause in particular—and which foods and nutrients have the exact opposite effect and should be avoided. At the same time, *how* to eat is just as important as what to eat. As menopause becomes more newsworthy, you'll see diets popping up left and right, claiming to tame it. Be cautious of these trends. They have little to do with menopause and everything to do with picking your pocket. Marketers jump at the chance to capitalize on our vulnerability as we dream of a flatter belly without the energy to obtain it. Some will go as far as to recommend you consume no more than 800 calories a day, advice that is not only unsustainable but reckless. One thing we've learned from decades of research is that diets based on extremes fail spectacularly in the end. Not only won't they deliver the promised results, but they often tamper with the delicate integrity of our bodies, brains, and hormones in the process. So I hope you're ready to throw some shade on ten-day cucumber cleanses, fad diets, and get-fit-quick ploys as we review the actual science on nutrition for menopause.

THE "GREENER" MEDITERRANEAN DIET

The best way to clarify which diets really work is to look at both science and tradition. Science speaks as to why particular diets work, while tradition lets us know if they've stood the test of time. When science meets tradition and the two agree, we're definitely on the right track.

Enter the Mediterranean diet.

Long praised as one of the world's healthiest diets, the traditional Mediterranean diet has well-documented protective effects on brain, heart, gut, and hormones—bestowing a reduced risk of heart disease, stroke, obesity, diabetes, cancer, depression, and dementia as compared to most other diets! When it comes to women's health in particular, the Mediterranean diet works like a charm, with positive effects on blood pressure, cholesterol, and blood glucose levels. As a result, women on a Mediterranean-style diet boast a 25 percent lower risk of heart attack and stroke than those following a Western-style diet high in processed foods, meat, sweets, and sugary beverages. Additionally, those who follow the Mediterranean diet in midlife have at least a 40 percent lower risk of developing depression in old age as compared to those on less healthy diets. They also have *half* the risk of breast cancer.

In more good news, women who follow a Mediterranean diet experience a generally milder menopause with far fewer hot flashes. For example, in a study of over 6,000 women who were experiencing menopausal symptoms, those who went on this diet experienced a 20 percent *decrease* in hot flashes and night sweats. Additionally, this diet pattern may *delay* the onset of menopause, too. A large examination of dietary data collected from 14,000 women revealed that consumption of legumes, like peas or beans, and fish is associated with a later onset of menopause by as many as three years. The other side of the story wasn't quite so pretty. Women who consumed less of these healthy foods and more processed foods and refined carbs like white rice and pasta exhibited an accelerated onset of menopause instead. These data also correlate with the fact that many women on a typical Western diet enter menopause early and suffer its effects more severely.

So how does the Mediterranean diet achieve such impressive benefits?

At a glance, it is low in calories and high in fiber, healthy fats, and complex carbohydrates—all key components of the nutrient-dense foods we discussed above. It contains no refined sugars or processed foods, a hallmark of good health we can't ignore. From a nutritional perspective, the Mediterranean diet is considered plant-centric, without being overly restrictive. Fresh vegetables and fruit, whole grains, legumes, and a variety of nuts and seeds are the stars of the show. Small amounts of seafood, eggs, or poultry are other typical entrées, while dairy and red meat are consumed sparingly and in moderation. Unrefined plant oils, like extra-virgin olive oil and flax oil, are the condiment of choice, paired with local vinegar or a squeeze of lemon juice. Bouquets of herbs and spices are used to flavor foods instead of table salt. Meals are often accompanied by a glass of red wine and finished off with a fragrant espresso—both rich sources of antioxidants. Desserts, including handmade pastries and artisanal gelato (made with high-quality ingredients), are not a daily event but are eaten with gusto on weekends or special occasions. The resulting combo platter is potent in antioxidants, polyphenols, fiber, and heart-healthy unsaturated fats—while allowing enough flexibility that one won't feel deprived.

Still, as potent as this diet can be, experts believe that a few tiny tweaks on the plan can make it even better for you. This healthy-fied Green Mediterranean diet further reduces the amount of meat on the menu and promotes plant-based protein instead, while introducing additional nutrient-dense foods that are not typically found in the Mediterranean region, such as green tea, avocados, and soybeans. This combination seems to amplify the benefits of the diet, leading to more fat loss around the midsection (the apple shape we discussed in the last chapter) and greater metabolic wins, as well as lower blood pressure, lower bad cholesterol, better insulin sensitivity, and less chronic inflammation. Additionally, while both dietary patterns slow the shrinkage of the hippocampus (that brain region that impacts our ability to learn and remember), the Green Mediterranean diet seems to offer potentially higher protection against aging and disease. While I'm not asking you to follow this diet to the letter, I would recommend trying this greener option, which we'll review below.

Before we begin, one of the many misconceptions regarding the Mediterranean diet is that it can be exclusive and/or expensive. I can assure you that this is not the case. The key is knowing what a *real* Mediterranean diet is, and not falling into the trap of all the inspired menus full of fancy ingredients, expensive wines and cheeses. The authentic Mediterranean diet is not expensive, by any standards. It involves local wine and seasonal produce, along with beans and whole grains as the main source of protein. As I mentioned earlier, meat and dairy—which are typically more expensive than produce—are more occasional indulgences. If you are interested in some tips on how to eat healthy without breaking the bank, I shared many in my first book, *Brain Food*. Here, the focus is on specific foods and nutrients that can be helpful with hormonal health and menopause. For some, most of these foods will be available at your local supermarket. For others, some foods may be difficult to come by or might be too expensive. In that case, simply swap them out for other options; this is more about a dietary approach than a strict plan or a shopping list. By focusing on a variety of plant-based whole foods, keeping an eye on your use of animal products, and staying away from ready-to-eat meals and processed foods, you'll improve your nutritional health in no time.

UP YOUR PLANT GAME

While you might be familiar with the old adage "Food is medicine," the truth is, *plants* are medicine. Plant foods are high in vitamins, minerals, and a bounty of *phytonutrients*, which help fight disease, reduce inflammation, and promote resilience throughout the entire body. Just as important, plants are the richest source of fiber, and fiber is the name of the game in women's health. In fact, some of the most potent nutritional advice I can deliver is to *eat enough fiber*.

Besides its positive effects on blood sugar, insulin levels, and digestion, fiber has the lesser-known skill of balancing estrogen levels. It facilitates the action of a molecule called *sex hormone binding globulin*, or SHBG, which regulates estrogen and testosterone levels in blood, effectively stacking hormones in our favor. As a result, eating enough fiber is a fantastic first-line defense against menopausal symptoms like hot flashes, which tend to be fewer and milder with fiber-rich diets. The balance fiber achieves in our bodies is essential for women in general, and for breast cancer survivors in particular. In the Women's Healthy Eating and Living Study, women treated for early stage breast cancer who consumed a high-fiber diet experienced a significant decrease in hot flashes in as little as one year. This study was only one among many showing clear-cut results. How much fiber is enough? As a rule of thumb, that's approximately 14 grams of fiber for each 1,000 calories you consume each day. For example, if you consume 2,000 calories per day for healthy weight maintenance, you should consume 28 grams of fiber.

Another big plus of eating more plant-based foods is that they offer some of the richest antioxidant choices available on the planet. Antioxidants fight off free radicals, reducing inflammation and delaying cellular aging. Since free radicals negatively affect egg maturation and release, while also wreaking havoc on your brain cells, a high intake of antioxidants may slow these effects, postponing menopause for longer. Among the mightiest antioxidants are vitamins C and E, beta-carotene, and the rare mineral selenium, along with a variety of phytonutrients, such as lycopene and anthocyanins, which grant blueberries, tomatoes, and grapes their beautiful red and blue hues. While you may think you know the top antioxidant-containing foods (let me guess . . . blueberries?), some might surprise you: blackberries, goji berries, and artichokes pack an even more powerful punch. Some spices and herbs, such as cinnamon, oregano, and rosemary, also compete, and citrus fruits famously show off in the vitamin C department. When it comes to selenium, Brazil nuts are a great source, but you can also find it in rice, oats, and lentils.

FRUIT AND VEG

Remember in the old-school cartoons when Popeye devoured his spinach straight from the can to flex rapid-fire muscles that saved the day? Although spinach alone may not accomplish miracles, eating more veggies may indeed do the trick.

Greens in particular are the foods least consumed in the standard Western diet, yet are the most essential for our health. Today, only one in every ten American adults consumes the minimum daily requirements for fruit or vegetables. In contrast, one in every two Americans eats *200 pounds* of red meat and poultry each year—and that's on top of all the processed foods consumed daily. Between these stats and those regarding lack of exercise, almost half of all U.S. adults will be obese by 2030. The rates of heart disease, stroke, and type 2 diabetes are also at an all-time high in many countries. Who's leading the pack? Sadly, women are winning that race, so we really need to pay closer attention to our food choices.

Many common chronic diseases are heavily impacted by diet, making it a no-brainer to optimize our foods in ways conducive to our health. To this end, most experts recommend we "eat the rainbow," consuming a wide array of colorful fruits and veggies at every meal. As a rule of thumb, vegetables should make up half of your plate in any given lunch or dinner. Among them, dark leafy greens and cruciferous vegetables are exceptionally conducive to hormonal balance and a healthy nervous system. For some examples, these include:

- *Leafy green vegetables:* kale, collard greens, spinach, cabbage, beet greens, watercress, romaine lettuce, Swiss chard, arugula, and endive.
- *Cruciferous vegetables:* cauliflower, broccoli, cabbage, kale, collard greens, mustard greens, garden cress, bok choy, Brussels sprouts.

Women who eat plenty of these veggie heroes have lower odds of being overweight or obese and far fewer menopausal symptoms than those who skip the veg and fill in the difference with fast food, processed foods, and commercially farmed meat and dairy. For instance, in a one-year intervention involving over 17,000 menopausal women, those eating more fiber-rich veggies, fruits, and beans experienced a 19 percent reduction in hot flashes compared with those who ate fewer plant-based foods. Likewise, a study of 393 postmenopausal women revealed that those eating more leafy greens and cruciferous vegetables had fewer menopausal symptoms while enjoying higher energy. Moreover, regular consumption of cruciferous vegetables may reduce damage to your genes, protecting you against breast cancer in turn. It is also associated with 50 percent lower odds of experiencing severe menopausal symptoms among breast cancer patients.

Let's not stop there. Low-to-medium glycemic vegetables like onions, beets, pumpkin, and carrots are also excellent choices, as is fruit. While some diets recommend avoiding fruit due to its sugar content, there's plenty of evidence that many fruits are uniquely beneficial to women's health and shouldn't be missed. In a study that followed 6,000 women for about nine years, those who ate fruit more regularly—

especially strawberries, pineapple, melons, apricots, and mangoes—had 20 percent fewer hot flashes and were in much better spirits compared with those who didn't eat as much fruit. Citrus fruit rich in antioxidant vitamin C, such as oranges, limes, lemons, grapefruit, and kumquats, also helped reduce a variety of symptoms. Another good reason to eat fruit: A study of over 16,000 women followed over many years showed that those who consumed flavonoid-rich berries, like blueberries and strawberries, had better cognitive performance than those who didn't. One or two servings of fresh fruit per day will do the trick. However, if you're particularly concerned about sugar, favor low-glycemic fruit like berries, apples, lemons, oranges, grapefruit, and watermelon—and eat higher-glycemic fruits like grapes and mangoes more sparingly.

WHOLE GRAINS, STARCHES, AND LEGUMES

While most people acknowledge that fruit and vegetables should be part of a healthy diet, there is debate over whether grains, potatoes, and legumes are friends or foes. Many have been taught to beware of carbs without realizing that not all carbs are created equally. In fact, carbohydrates can be simple or complex based on how much fiber, starch, and sugar they contain. Foods containing more fiber than sugar are typically called complex carbs and have a lower glycemic load. As a result, they are gentler on the body, slowly releasing their natural sugars, which are readily metabolized into energy without causing spikes in your insulin levels. Whole grains (those with the husk still on) like brown rice, wheat berries, and steel-cut oats, as well as most legumes and tubers like sweet potatoes, fall in this complex carb category, explaining why they are also referred to as "good" carbs. From a women's health perspective, eating low-glycemic carbs has been linked to very favorable outcomes, such as a markedly lowered risk of heart disease, type 2 diabetes, depression, and dementia—not to mention better sleep!

On the other end of the spectrum are high-glycemic carbs, possessing a high dose of sugar, likely refined sugar at that, and little to no fiber. These foods, sometimes labeled "bad" carbs, trigger spikes in blood sugar levels, making it hard for your body's insulin to metabolize so much quick sugar at once. Over time, this exhausts your pancreas, causing insulin resistance. Insulin resistance inflames your body and its systems, posing a risk factor for metabolic disorders, diabetes, and heart disease. It can also harm estrogen production, the last thing anyone needs. Great examples of high-glycemic carbs aren't just the obvious ones like packaged treats, sugary cookies, commercial pastries, and candies. The high-sugar carb club has numerous members, including sodas, sweetened drinks, and processed grains such as sandwich bread, white bread, white rice, commercial pasta, bagels, and rolls.

Folks, the jury's in. If we want to optimize our health as women, whole grains and legumes are in; refined grains are out. Sweet potatoes and regular potatoes with the skin on are also in; processed potato-based products and French fries from McDonald's are out. You get the idea.

For those who avoid gluten, naturally gluten-free whole grains such as rice (brown, red, black), wild rice (technically a seed), quinoa (also a seed), amaranth, buckwheat, millet, sorghum, and teff are legitimate sources of good carbs. But beware of the many gluten-free products masquerading as healthy alternatives while they're nothing more than yet another processed junk food.

NATURAL SWEETENERS

We'd all do well to ditch white sugar and artificial sweeteners once and for all. Natural unrefined ones like raw honey, maple syrup, stevia, and coconut sugar are a whole other thing. Richer in vitamins and minerals than the powdery or granular white stuff, these sweeteners are gentler on the body and don't pound as hard at your blood sugar levels.

If you, like me, can't function without the occasional treat, I strongly recommend dark chocolate with a cacao content of 80 percent or higher. Or better yet, try *raw* dark chocolate. In its purest form, this type of chocolate is a powerful superfood with an impressive health pedigree. It has a low glycemic load, is satisfying without a sugar crash, and it's rich in theobromine, a kick-ass antioxidant. Also packing powerful *flavonols* that combat inflammation and estrogen-supporting *catechins*, raw chocolate is a welcome treat. For some inspiration, I am going to share one of my all-time favorite recipes: a delicious three-ingredient dark chocolate ganache. Begin by melting ½ cup of unsweetened dark chocolate chips and ¼ cup of unrefined coconut oil. Then stir in 1 heaping tablespoon of raw cacao powder and a tablespoon of maple syrup. Pour the mixture into an airtight container and freeze for about three hours. This dessert not only provides a burst of energy but also a healthy dose of antioxidants, making it a delightful and guilt-free indulgence.

FEED YOUR ESTROBOLOME

Here's another impressive yet poorly publicized benefit of eating more plants. It's become common knowledge that our bodies are host to trillions of bacteria called the *microbiome*, chiefly residing in our gastrointestinal tract. Scientific research has demonstrated that these gut microbes help regulate many aspects of our physiology, including nutrient absorption, intestinal strength, and immunity. However, few are aware those same microbes also play nice with our precious estrogen.

Meet the estrobolome, a widely overlooked collection of gut bacteria with the unique ability of metabolizing estrogen. Here's how it works: Once estrogen makes its rounds throughout the body, spreading its magic, it heads for the intestines, where it's either reabsorbed into the bloodstream or eliminated the same way nutrients are. The estrobolome is in charge of this process. These bacteria produce an enzyme called *beta-glucuronidase*, which breaks down estrogen into its active forms, deciding whether to send it back in the circulation or pass it out of the system. By making this call, the estrobolome keeps things in balance, ensuring that the overall amount of estrogen in the body is just right. Moreover, the estrobolome is an expert at breaking down complex carbs and putting antioxidants to work, which further underscores the connection between estrogen and plant-based foods.

Taking good care of these friendly bacteria pays off, keeping us all healthy campers. A top-drawer gut is associated with a lower risk of obesity, heart disease, dementia, depression, cancer, and a gentler menopause. The opposite is also true. If you're already gut savvy, you may have heard of *dysbiosis*—a problem that arises when gut microbes are outnumbered by harmful bacteria and knocked out of balance. Dysbiosis results in digestive issues and overall inflammation, making our estrobolome . . . *estrobummed*. As a result, estrogen levels may also be out of whack, resulting in jagged levels being released in the bloodstream.

What causes dysbiosis? While chronic stress and overusing antibiotics play their parts, a poor diet is the biggest culprit. Your estrobolome, as well as your entire microbiome, goes to town on plants—the more, the merrier. When you eat a wide variety of plant-based foods, your microbiome receives the bounty of nutrients on which it relies. Avoiding processed foods and reducing meat and dairy also seems to help, as people who follow diets high in fiber and low in animal fat boast the healthiest microbiomes. Consider this: Eating processed foods *for as little as two weeks* can reduce the biodiversity of your microbiome by 40 percent and, at the same time, put your estrogen-balancing bacteria in jeopardy and your health with it. Our society's tendency to go on diets low in fiber and high in low-quality nutrients is wreaking havoc on us, like it or not. Fortunately, there is a foolproof way to restore our microbiome. You guessed it: eating more plants mends the mess. To restore your gut bacteria, focus on foods rich in *prebiotics, probiotics,* and the lesser-known *bitters*:

- *Prebiotics* are nondigestible carbohydrates, your gut bacteria's favorite menu. Garlic, onions, asparagus, beets, cabbage, leeks, and artichokes are fantastic sources, as are legumes like beans, peas, and lentils.
- *Probiotics* are live bacteria that repopulate the microbiome. Find these in fermented foods like sauerkraut, kimchi, unsweetened yogurt, and brine-fermented pickles. Probiotic supplements can also be helpful, especially those containing at least three different strains: lactobacillus, rhamnosus, and bifidobacterium.
- *Bitters* are a group of plants that are defined by exactly what their name implies: their bitterness. Bitter herbs like dandelion greens, endive, radicchio, and arugula are powerful digestive stimulants that love up the microbiome. Toss these veggies with lemon juice or vinegar for maximum benefits.

THE CASE FOR PHYTOESTROGENS

Estrogen is an ancient hormone that we produce as humans. However, it is not unique to us, as many other animals and plants make it, too. Case in point, scientists have identified almost 300 plants that produce *phytoestrogen*, or plant-based estrogen, similar in its chemical makeup to the estrogen made by our ovaries and with similar functionalities. Now, there is some confusion over what phytoestrogens can and can't do for women's health. Some people believe that phytoestrogens pump up estrogen levels, calling them fertility heroes, while others declare them villains that render you potentially prone to certain cancers (which is how soy got a bad rep). Others still regard phytoestrogens as ineffective or useless. The internet weighs in, some sites claiming you shouldn't consume them at all to avoid developing estrogen dominance. I could write a treatise on this topic, but I figured you might appreciate the quicker Q&A that follows.

Which Foods Contain Phytoestrogens?

There are three main types of phytoestrogens:

- *Isoflavones* are found in soybeans, tofu, tempeh, lima beans, chickpeas, and lentils.
- *Lignans* are found in seeds like flaxseed and sesame; fruits such as dried apricots, dates, peaches, and berries; and vegetables like garlic, winter squash, and green beans. They are also in grains such as wheat and rye and nuts like pistachios and almonds.
- *Coumestans* are found in sprouting seeds such as alfalfa.

Do Phytoestrogens Have Any Effects on the Human Body?

Phytoestrogens have a molecular structure similar to that of the estrogen produced by our ovaries, and they bind to the same receptors. As such, they function similarly to our own estrogen but are weaker. Their ability to latch on to estrogen receptors is only a thousandth of the strength of estradiol. As a result, their effects are much milder, unless you combine them together in specific amounts. In this case, their activity is amplified. Nonetheless, these foods have an effect only when consumed consistently. (In case you're wondering, no, phytoestrogens won't stop your body from making its own estrogen.)

Are Phytoestrogens Dangerous?

On the contrary, these compounds show a protective role in hormonal health. Phytoestrogens are peculiar compounds. They carry out both estrogenic and anti-estrogenic activities and are selective in their application. In fact, they are very similar to the selective estrogen receptor modulators, or SERMs, used for cancer treatment. While the exact mechanisms of their action are still under investigation, phytoestrogens tend to adjust to the estrogen level in your bloodstream and may be in cahoots with the estrobolome in your gut. When estrogen levels are high enough, phytoestrogens may gently block estrogen receptors, protecting you from excess exposure. When estrogen levels are low, phytoestrogens may step in to bolster those levels, though in a much milder way than your own estrogen.

Can Phytoestrogens, Soy in Particular, Cause Cancer?

Soy is one of the most controversial foods on the planet. You will find it promoted as a superfood one minute and listed as a cancer-inducing poison the next. However, Asian women eat soy regularly and are four times *less likely* to get breast cancer than their Western counterparts. While genetic and cultural factors also play a role, many studies have shown a lower rate of breast cancer in populations consuming soy as a regular part of the diet. These women are less likely to suffer from hot flashes, osteoporosis, and heart disease, too. At the very least, that's an indication that soy is unlikely to be dangerous.

Overall, there is no evidence that soy or the phytoestrogens it carries cause cancer. For many years, professional societies recommended avoiding soy and other estrogenic plants. However, more rigorous research led both the American Institute for Cancer Research and the American Cancer Society to revise their position in 2013. Today, soy is considered safe for women, including patients with breast cancer. Extensive research has shown that soy does not increase the odds of breast tumor recurrence and, in some cases, may even reduce mortality. Additionally, soy has no adverse effects on endometrial, ovarian, or other cancers.

One caveat: People who are allergic to soy should avoid both soy and its derivatives. Also, the type of soy you're eating matters. The traditional soy products consumed in Asia are clean, unprocessed, and often fermented, which most of our soy is not. In the Western world, most soy products are made of genetically modified soybeans rife with pesticides and preservatives. Worse yet, processed soybean oil, soy lecithin, and isolated soy protein lace everything from packaged foods and breakfast cereals to lattes and infant formulas—and have nothing to do with good health. Stay clear of considering these versions of soy as anything resembling a superfood. If you are interested in eating soy to support a healthy menopause, seek organic and fermented soy, such as fresh edamame, miso, and tempeh.

Are There Benefits to Eating Phytoestrogens?

While the findings are not always consistent, clinical trials indicate that eating soy and, more generally, isoflavones potentially lessens the number of hot flashes. In a recent study published by the North American Menopause Society, a plant-based diet rich in soy reduced moderate to severe hot flashes by as much as 84 percent, lowering a five-a-day occurrence to fewer than once a day. In this study, postmenopausal women experiencing hot flashes were randomly assigned to a plant-based diet, including half a cup of cooked soybeans added to a salad or soup each day. The remaining participants made up the control group and were given no dietary changes. During the twelve-week study, over half of participants on the plant-based, soy-enriched diet became *free* of hot flashes. Most participants also reported an improved quality of life, mood, libido, and overall energy. Although this was a small study, the results are impressive, meriting consideration.

FOCUS ON ESSENTIAL FATS

Just like carbohydrates, not all fat is created equal. While for many years, people were advised to reduce the overall quantity of fat in the diet, it turns out that the type of fat is more important than the actual amount being consumed. There are three main kinds of fat, each with its distinct effects:

- *Unsaturated fat* can be *monounsaturated*, as in olive oil and avocado) or *polyunsaturated*, found in fish, shellfish, and various nuts and seeds, as well as some vegetables, grains, and legumes.

- *Saturated fat* is abundant in dairy, meat, and certain oils (like coconut oil).
- *Trans-unsaturated fats, or trans fats,* are produced when unsaturated oils are processed using a procedure called hydrogenation. This makes them become similar to saturated fats, achieving a longer shelf life. These trans fats typically lurk in processed foods and are the worst fat you can eat, so much so that they're banned in many countries. We'll discuss them later in "Foods to Avoid."

Omega-3s Are the Real Stars

Much women-based research reveals that polyunsaturated fat supports women's health, showing a reduced risk of heart disease, obesity, diabetes, and dementia. These female-friendly fats come in different varieties, the most common being omega-3 and omega-6 fatty acids. Omega-3s are particularly helpful thanks to their anti-inflammatory and antioxidant effects. In contrast, women who don't consume enough omega-3s may experience more menstrual pain, fertility issues, and postpartum as well as menopausal depression.

There are different types of omega-3s:

- *ALA, or alpha-linolenic acid,* found exclusively in plant foods.
- *EPA, or eicosapentaenoic acid,* and *DHA, or docosahexaenoic acid,* found mainly in fish and seafood, but also seaweed and algae.

ALA, EPA, and DHA are all referred to as essential fats because the body cannot produce them on its own and you can obtain them only by eating the proper foods. However, ALA is the only omega-3 that's *literally* essential. That's because the body can use ALA to make the other two, EPA and DHA. However, quite a bit of ALA is lost in the process, so it's important to be mindful of this.

Most dietary guidelines for women recommend getting at least 1,100 mg of omega-3s every day. This dosage is easily achieved, for example, by using flaxseed (linseed) oil. This beautiful golden oil is made from flaxseeds that have been ground and pressed to release their natural oil. Just one tablespoon (15 ml) contains an impressive 7,200 mg of omega-3 ALA, so you're set for the day. Other excellent alternatives include ground flaxseed, hempseed, walnuts, and almonds. Olives, olive oil, avocados, and soybeans are also excellent sources, as are broccoli, sweet peas, and many leafy greens. Algae and seaweed are important sources of omega-3s for people on vegan or vegetarian diets, or anyone who doesn't eat fish, as they are one of the few plant foods containing preassembled DHA and EPA.

Monounsaturated Fat Makes Your Heart Happy

Monounsaturated fat is known for its protective effects on heart health. Nuts like almonds, pistachios, Brazil nuts, cashews, and hazelnuts are high in monounsaturated fat, as are fatty fruits like avocados and olives, and some seeds like sesame and sunflower. In a study of over 86,000 women, those who frequently consumed nuts had a much lower risk of heart disease and stroke. A handful of nuts or seeds (about an ounce) once a week, with the peel still on, delivers targeted results. Avoid blanched, flavored, salted, sweetened, or seasoned nuts and seeds. This snack is often mistaken for healthy, but it's processed and laden with chemicals and sugars.

Saturated Fat Is Best from Plant-Based Sources

Saturated fat comes from both animal sources, such as meat and dairy, and plant-based sources, like coconuts, avocados, and nuts, such as cashews and macadamia nuts. There is increasing evidence that saturated *vegetable* fat supports women's health through its beneficial effects on our hormones, while saturated fat from animal sources does not show the same result. A possible explanation is that vegetable fat seems to have a gentler impact on blood lipid levels than animal fat. For example, in randomized clinical trials, dairy butter increased LDL cholesterol significantly, whereas olive oil and coconut oil did not. To be clear, we are referring to vegetable fat derived from whole foods, and not from products like margarine or processed plant-based spreads.

Too much animal fat has also been linked to an increased risk of hormone-related cancers. In the Nurses' Health Study, women who consumed more animal products, especially red meat and high-fat dairy, had three times the risk of developing breast cancer compared with those who consumed fewer of these foods. This could be because animal fat, contrary to fiber, has negative effects on the estrogen-balancing SHBG molecule. Possibly as a result, replacing some animal fat with vegetable fat, especially oils high in antioxidants like extra-virgin olive oil and flaxseed oil, has been linked to a reduced risk of breast cancer, heart disease, and diabetes in women.

Cholesterol Is Important for Hormonal Health

Cholesterol often gets a bad rap, but in truth, this type of fat plays a crucial role in many bodily functions, from forming healthy cell walls to making enough estrogen. However, too much of certain types of cholesterol can get you in trouble. There are different kinds of cholesterol:

- HDL (high-density lipoprotein), aka "good" cholesterol.
- LDL (low-density lipoprotein) and VLDL (very low-density lipoprotein), which are considered "bad" cholesterol. High levels of bad cholesterol have been linked to plaque buildup in the arteries and other heart issues, too.

Measuring your cholesterol levels is an effective way to determine your risk of heart disease and stroke. There are two ways to do this.

One way is to measure your total cholesterol. Typically, you want this number to be below 200. An even better way is to calculate your cholesterol ratio. The latter will give you a breakdown of your good vs. bad cholesterol, delivering a clearer picture of your health. If your total cholesterol is 200 and your HDL cholesterol is 50, your ratio is 4. A ratio lower than 4.5 is considered good, but 2 or 3 is best.

If your cholesterol is above limits, it's important to lower it. Cholesterol comes from two sources: Some 80 percent or so is made by the liver, while the rest comes from the foods you eat. Traditionally, doctors advised their patients to reduce their consumption of cholesterol-rich foods, especially eggs, to lower their cholesterol levels. However, newer research has shown that cholesterol from food doesn't raise the cholesterol in the blood nearly as much as other types of fats do, chiefly trans fats and saturated fats from animal sources, so that's another reason to avoid or reduce those other fats. Eating more plants is also helpful in this regard because plants simply don't contain any cholesterol to start with. Some multitasking plant-based foods can also help lower your bad LDL while at the same time promoting the production of good HDL. These include avocados, lemons, oranges, beans, legumes, and whole grains like oats and brown rice. Cooking and seasoning with fruit oils (such as olive and coconut oils) rather than butter or animal fats also fit the bill.

LEAN PROTEIN

The word *protein* often conjures up images of bodybuilders and dumbbells. But this macronutrient is so much more than that. In fact, protein is a critical building block that our bodies use in a multitude of ways, from making new cells and repairing damaged ones to being a component of many hormones. Protein also keeps our bones sturdy by maintaining a process known as bone remodeling, thus reducing the risk of osteoporosis. Further, a diet including adequate amounts of protein combined with regular exercise works to regenerate muscle mass. So eating adequate protein during menopause can help keep our metabolism running smoothly while supporting a healthy weight.

As with the carbs and fats, protein comes in many types. The one we want to prioritize is high-quality lean protein. Lean protein is typically lower in saturated fat and therefore calories—hence the word *lean*. It is found in a wide variety of foods of animal origin, such as fish, poultry, and lean meat cuts, as well as a variety of foods of plant origin, which we'll discuss in greater detail below. First, let's address the common concern that diets rich in plant foods may lack sufficient protein.

Protein is made up of chains of molecules known as amino acids. There are twenty amino acids found in nature that your body uses to build protein. Out of these, nine are considered essential. Remember, *essential* means that your body cannot produce these nutrients on its own, so you need to eat them in your diet. Protein of animal origin contains all nine essential amino acids, typically in sufficient amounts per portion. As such, it's referred to as complete protein. Plants also contain these essential amino acids, though typically have a limited amount of at least one of them. For instance, vegetables and legumes tend to contain low amounts of cysteine and methionine. Grains, nuts, and seeds tend to be lacking in lysine. Because of this, many people refer to plant foods as incomplete protein. However, as long as you eat a variety of plant-based foods, you can easily tally up sufficient amounts of essential amino acids by combining different plant foods in the same meal. The renowned rice and beans combo is a good example. Besides, some plant foods actually contain more protein per portion than some animal products. For example, green peas, which are actually part of the bean family. Believe it or not, a cup of these yummy peas has more protein than a cup of milk. For another honorable mention, spirulina (a type of blue-green algae) contains 8 grams of *complete* protein per just 2 tablespoons of the green stuff. Nutritional yeast, a common vegan cheese substitute, also delivers 8 grams of complete protein in just half a tablespoon. I am not suggesting you consume these foods if you don't enjoy them. Rather, the aim is to clarify that plant-based foods are viable sources of protein. Returning to our starting point, if you eat animal foods, fish, eggs, and poultry are readily found sources of lean protein. Plant foods that contain a good amount of lean protein per serving include:

- seitan (25 grams of protein per 3.5 ounces, or 100 grams)
- tofu, tempeh, and edamame (12–20 grams per 3.5 ounces, or 100 grams)
- lentils (18 grams per cooked cup, or 170 grams)
- beans (15 grams per cooked cup)
- spelt and teff (10–11 grams per cooked cup, or 250 grams), making these ancient grains higher in protein than quinoa
- quinoa (8–9 grams per cooked cup, or 185 grams)
- green peas (9 grams per cooked cup, or 160 grams)
- spirulina (8 grams of complete protein per 2 tablespoons)
- hempseed (9 grams per 3 tablespoons)
- oats (5 grams of protein per ½ cup of dry oats)

IRON

Iron is another concern that often pops up when considering a plant-focused diet. Plant foods contain a type of iron called *non-heme iron*, which is generally less bioavailable (less easily absorbed by the body) than the iron found in meat, called *heme iron*. So the problem is not simply the quantity of iron present in the foods but our bodies' ability to absorb it. In fact, many plant foods are perfectly good sources of iron, including oats, soybeans, legumes, and leafy greens. Some of these foods contain even more iron than meat. For example, 3 cups of spinach or 1 cup of lentils have more iron than an 8-ounce steak. However, their iron is not as promptly put to good use. One way to increase the absorption of plant iron is to combine these foods with other foods rich in vitamin C. For example, sprinkle some berries on your oats or lemon juice into your salads and, *voilà!* mission accomplished.

VITAMIN B$_{12}$

Vitamin B$_{12}$ is the only vitamin you can't obtain from plants. In this case, eating a flexible diet that contains B$_{12}$ or taking a supplement is in order. That said, even with a proper diet, many people over the age of fifty may need vitamin B$_{12}$ supplements to make sure they're hitting the recommended intake. According to the National Institutes of Health (NIH), up to 43 percent of older adults suffer from a B$_{12}$ deficiency. More on this in chapter 15.

CALCIUM-RICH FOODS

It is no big secret that we need more calcium and vitamin D to support bone health as we age. But contrary to popular belief, you don't need dairy to get calcium; many plant-based foods are just as good. Various vegetables pack a punch, like spinach, turnips, kale, bok choy, and mustard greens, as well as legumes like soybeans, tofu, beans, and peas. Seeds can be good sources, too. Consider this: A glass of whole milk contains about 280 milligrams of calcium, as does 1 cup of cooked spinach or 2 tablespoons of tahini. Another easy way to swap out animal-based for plant-based calcium is by drinking plant-based milk; many of these beverages have roughly the same amount of calcium as cow-dairy.

Vitamin D is difficult to obtain from diet alone, no matter what you eat. It's not called the "sunshine vitamin" for nothing. Our bodies manufacture vitamin D from cholesterol when our skin is exposed to the sun. Get your vitamin D levels checked, and if they're low, you've got a doc's note to book that tropical vacation you've always wanted!

Otherwise, stock up on foods fortified with vitamin D or take a supplement (discussed in the next chapter).

A final note on dairy products. There is a great deal of conjecture that the hormonal residues in dairy from growth factors fed to dairy cows may contribute to tumor growth in humans, though this has not been thoroughly researched. While the jury is still out on the role of dairy products on breast cancer, focusing on organic dairy free of growth hormone is important should you choose to consume it. Goat or sheep milk is also more easily digestible than cow's milk.

MELATONIN FOR SLEEP SUPPORT

Believe it or not, some foods contain melatonin, the sleep-cuing hormone. Pistachios in particular are the most melatonin-rich food on the planet. Eating a whole handful of pistachios is equivalent to popping a melatonin supplement before bed. This shell-snapping snack is also a great source of fiber, vitamin B_6, and some essential amino acids. Melatonin can also be found in some mushrooms, especially the portobello variety, as well as various sprouted seeds and lentils. Wheat, barley, and oats are also good sources, as are grapes, dark cherries, and strawberries. Imagine a dinner salad garnished with sprouted lentils, roasted mushrooms, and pistachios—with a strawberry sorbet for dessert. Your estrobolome will love you for it, and perhaps you won't have to count sheep that night.

FOODS TO AVOID

Whenever someone asks me for my number one diet tip for brain health, I always, without fail, give the same answer: *do not eat processed foods*. People in the United States, Canada, and the UK consume almost 50 percent of their daily calories from processed foods, many of which are not only processed but *ultra*-processed. That means nearly half of the food we eat daily has been *significantly* modified from its original state, with the most detrimental versions of salt, sugars, fats, additives, preservatives, and artificial colors and flavors. Ultra-processed foods undergo multiple processes (extrusion, molding, milling, and so forth), contain long lists of added chemicals, and are highly manipulated. Examples are commercial white bread loaves, packaged pastries, snacks, and all industrialized confectionery and desserts; commercially fried and prepared foods; and all fast food, including but not limited to soft drinks, soda, and sugar-sweetened beverages; processed meat and cold cuts; processed cheeses; margarine, shortening, and lard; instant noodles and soups; frozen or shelf-stable meals; most bottled condiments, spreads, and creamers; chips, chocolate, candy, ice cream, sweetened breakfast cereals, packaged soups, chicken nuggets, burgers, hot dogs, and so forth (the list, unfortunately, could fill its own book). Depending on where you're shopping, supermarkets may carry more processed and ultra-processed foods than minimally or unprocessed foods. In chapter 17, we'll go over specific tips to recognize and avoid the toxic ingredients in these foods.

For now, suffice it to say that the more ultra-processed foods you eat, the poorer the overall nutritional quality of your diet, and the poorer your health. The World Cancer Research Fund and the American Institute for Cancer Research state that ultra-processed foods may well cause one-third of all the world's cancers. Processed foods, such as salty snacks and processed meat in particular, have also been identified as the culprit behind an estimated 45 percent of deaths from heart disease, stroke, and diabetes. After evaluating over 800 studies, the World Health Organization (WHO) concluded that processed meat is also carcinogenic, much like tobacco smoking and asbestos. Processed meat is meat that is salted, cured, fermented, smoked, or otherwise processed to enhance flavor and improve preservation, such as most lunch meats sold at your deli counter, supermarket, or sandwich shop. These meats include commercial boiled ham, roast beef, turkey, chicken, bologna, and hot dogs.

CUT DOWN ON ALCOHOL, CAFFEINE, AND SPICY FOODS

Navigating the culinary landscape of menopause can be quite the adventure. It's no secret that certain foods—chiefly spicy foods, alcohol, and caffeine in coffee, tea, or energy drinks—have a knack for aggravating those pesky symptoms. As every woman is different, it's important to play detective with your taste buds and notice whether these foods trigger or worsen any symptoms you have, and experiment with reducing or avoiding these foods and drinks.

Generally, spicy foods can contribute to the sensation of heat rising in your body or make your hot flashes perform an encore. Alcohol is also famous for worsening hot flashes. While many think a drink may help them fall asleep, it may be the culprit behind your midnight wake-up call. Additionally, while red wine can still have its cardio-protective charms in a 5-ounce glass per day, moderation is key to keep the breast cancer risk at bay.

Now, let's talk caffeine. As much as many of us adore the morning java jolt, it's worth noting that caffeine can be a double troublemaker—it can make hot flashes worse while also having negative effects on sleep. Caffeine can take up to twelve hours to leave your system, so why not limit yourself to one cup per day, savored before noon? Here's an interesting twist: contrary to popular belief, freshly brewed espresso can actually be gentler on your menopausal woes compared to an Americano. The shorter extraction time of espresso means it contains less caffeine than its diluted counterpart. You can thank me later!

SERIOUSLY, DRINK WATER

When it comes to what drink is the healthiest, the best advice I can give you is to drink *water*. Given how critical water is for the brain, I dedicated an entire chapter to this remarkable nutrient in *Brain Food*.

Moreover, proper hydration is just as crucial for hormonal health and menopause. Here's a brief overview:

- Even *mild* dehydration can trigger dizziness, confusion, fatigue, and big-time brain fog, at any age. Keeping hydrated reduces the risk of all these symptoms, which are common in menopause.
- Staying hydrated can help support the body's hormone production and balance.
- Proper hydration helps to regulate body temperature, helping to lessen hot flashes.
- Proper hydration is also key to vaginal lubrication, which comes in handy after menopause.
- Drinking water aids in digestion, circulation, and elimination, ensuring the body can function optimally and fight inflammation.
- Hydration is crucial for maintaining healthy joints, reducing discomfort and stiffness.
- Drinking water helps keep the skin and hair hydrated, promoting elasticity and reducing dryness.

This may sound weird, but the type and quality of water actually matters. See, water isn't just water. Our bodies, brains, and hormonal systems don't just need something *wet*. We specifically need natural water, complete with its native minerals, salts, and electrolytes. Drinking spring water, mineral water, or filtered tap water that retains its electrolytes is the best way to support hydration. Purified water, club soda, and seltzer don't cut it, since they don't contain any of the hydrating nutrients that *actual* water does. Soda (Coke or other similar beverages) is not water in the first place, and can do a number on your ovaries, as it's associated with an increased risk of ovulatory infertility.

Another smart way to support hydration is to *eat your water*. An ounce of water-rich fruits or vegetables is equivalent to an ounce of water trapped in a web of nutrients—fiber, phytonutrients, and antioxidants. Think radishes, watermelon, cucumbers, strawberries, tomatoes, watercress, apples, celery, melons, lettuce, peaches, and cauliflower—these fruits and vegetables are quick to quench!

EAT MINDFULLY

The obesity epidemic has spawned an entire industry of weight-loss programs. Currently getting a lot of attention is intermittent fasting, which broadly involves alternating intervals of eating and not eating, or eating fewer calories at specific times. This may help shed pounds and stabilize weight more efficiently than other types of diets, while also reducing inflammation and risk of heart disease. As a result, intermittent fasting is often also recommended for menopausal women.

Here's my take on this. First, while there is rigorous research behind time-restricted feeding in laboratory animals, scientific evidence for the health benefits of intermittent fasting *in humans* is more limited than you may think. Research studies in people have small sample sizes and focus on very specific populations, mainly overweight individuals with or without diabetes or well-trained athletes. Second, there are several trendy versions of this practice that have nothing to do with science. Instead, they come out of people's personal opinions about what one should eat and not eat to break the fast or throughout the rest of the day. Many of these plans border on nonsense. Just as important, research on intermittent fasting in women is still relatively limited compared to studies involving men. Even less work has been done concerning this practice during menopause, not even in animals, so better be wary of the headlines.

In many parts of the world, there is a form of "fasting" that's been around for centuries, if not millennia, and is both doable and sensible. It's called . . . sleeping. The world's healthiest dietary patterns all involve having a light dinner early in the evening, and then refraining from eating overnight, which is when you should be winding down and sleeping instead. Once you get up the day after, usually ten to twelve hours later, you have a proper breakfast and are ready to go on with your day.

In the end, the only successful diets—whatever the goal—involve sustainable and long-lasting changes in eating habits that are conducive to health. I'd argue that how we approach our food is just as important, if not more so, than a specific eating schedule. Making smart food choices and eating mindfully throughout the day are both key in this respect. Mindful eating stems from the broader philosophy of mindfulness, a widespread centuries-old practice in many cultures and religions. Eating mindfully means using your physical and emotional senses to experience and enjoy your food choices. This focus encourages options that are both satisfying *and* nourishing. Most of us are busy, rushed, and poised over our keyboards as we gobble our meals. What if we slowed down and paid better attention? When we do, we know when we're *genuinely* physically hungry as opposed to having eaten enough. This also helps to alleviate digestive upset like bloating and heartburn, your body's way of avenging that spicy calzone you inhaled in seventeen seconds flat. As most people in Western countries tend to overeat to start with, paying more attention to the moment-to-moment experience of eating can help improve the quality of your diet, too. This consciousness in turn may allow us to manage cravings more efficiently, reduce stress-eating, and lose weight when necessary.

In conclusion, when it comes to dietary choices during menopause, the key is to focus on a balanced, nutritious, and sustainable approach. Instead of falling for fad diets or restrictive eating patterns, prioritize consuming whole foods, proper hydration, and plenty of plants. Incorporating a variety of fruits, vegetables, whole grains, lean protein, and healthy fats is key to providing the necessary nutrients to support your hormonal health and overall well-being. While it's important to be mindful of portion sizes and caloric intake, it's equally important to listen to your body's hunger and fullness cues. Avoid overly strict or rigid approaches that may lead to feelings of deprivation or disrupt a healthy relationship with food. Remember, there is no one-size-fits-all approach to nutrition during menopause. By embracing a sensible approach to eating, you can nourish your body, brain, and hormones throughout the menopausal transition and beyond, keeping your inner thermostat in check and your zest for life vibrant.

15

Supplements and Botanicals

THE POWER OF PLANTS

While HRT has long been a standard treatment for menopausal symptoms, concerns about its risks have made for a history of fits and starts. These stumbles, combined with a renaissance of interest in herbal remedies and supplements for hormonal health, produced a dramatic increase in so-called natural solutions. As a result, up to half of all women in industrialized countries now rely on plant-based supplements for menopause.

Generally, supplements can be divided into *botanicals* (like soy extracts, black cohosh, and ginseng) and *non-botanicals* (such as vitamins and minerals). Botanicals are often divided into having and not having estrogenic effects, which makes the latter more suitable for women with concerns about breast cancer. From ancient times to the present day, every culture around the world has employed a variety of plants as the basis for their medicinal needs. Several types of herbs have been used to manage hot flashes, including black cohosh, dong quai, evening primrose, ginseng, flaxseed, red clover, St. John's wort, and wild yam. Other botanicals, such as maca and horny goat weed, are used to boost sex drive, while lemon balm, valerian, and passionflower are often recommended for the insomnia, anxiety, and fatigue that can accompany the transition. However, while some of these preparations are supported by scientific evidence, others are not. For example, wild yam creams used to soothe hot flashes show no effect in clinical studies, whereas phytoestrogen supplements (a more concentrated, potent version of the phytoestrogens present in our foods) figure prominently as having positive effects. Ideally, one would want to try out the latter and avoid the former, so check out my notes to each supplement.

A word of caution before we begin. Many people attempt to employ supplements as shortcuts, sidestepping dietary demands, and are upset when supplements fail to achieve their goals. So keep in mind that nutritional supplements are *complementary* in nature and cannot replace a healthy diet or lifestyle.

Another consideration is that supplements are not subject to the scrutiny of federal regulatory bodies like the FDA. Unlike prescription drugs, they provide no guarantee of efficacy or safety. Since they're not regulated, there is also no double check to ascertain the supplement contains the indicated amount of active ingredients listed. Because of this, selecting *standardized* formulations is imperative. To make sure a formula is standardized, you'll want to check the *percentage* of active ingredients listed. For example, when searching for a ginkgo biloba supplement, you want to be sure extracts are standardized to contain a certain percentage (typically 25 percent) of ginkgo flavone glycosides, the herb's active constituents.

Another way to ensure a dietary supplement is of high, uncontaminated quality is to purchase products indicating testing by either the U.S. Pharmacopeial (USP) Convention Dietary Supplement Verification Program or ConsumerLab.com. Finally, while most supplements and herbal remedies carry a low risk of side effects, some can interact with prescription medications or come with contraindications, as noted below.

Botanicals

▶ **BLACK COHOSH**

Black cohosh (*Actaea racemosa, Cimicifuga racemosa*) belongs to the North American buttercup family and is one of the most extensively researched herbs for menopause. Native American women have used black cohosh for centuries to relieve menstrual cramps and menopausal symptoms. Clinical trials have examined this herb with about half reporting decreases in hot flashes, which is not considered a consistent effect. Nonetheless, this buttercup seems to specialize in soothing mild to moderate night sweats and mood swings. In Germany, black cohosh is approved for premenstrual discomfort and menopausal symptoms such as hot flashes, heart palpitations, nervousness, irritability, disturbed sleep, vertigo, and depression.

Although more research is needed, black cohosh doesn't appear to have estrogenic effects. As such, it may be helpful for cancer patients.

Usage: Hot flashes.

Scientific proof of efficacy: Medium.

Dosage: 40 mg per day of standardized extract. Due to the lack of long-term safety studies, it should be used for a maximum of six months.

Precautions: Although black cohosh is generally well tolerated, it can cause headaches. Rare cases of liver damage have been reported.

▶ **CHASTE TREE BERRY**

Contrary to what its name suggests, chaste tree berry (*Vitex agnus-castus*) is often recommended to boost fertility and improve some symptoms of menopause. However, while chaste tree berry seems to have hormone-balancing effects, clinical trials have yet to show consistent relief of menopause symptoms.

Usage: Menopausal complaints of various origin.

Scientific proof of efficacy: Low.

Dosage: 200–250 mg per day.

Precautions: Generally well tolerated. It may interact with some medicines, such as birth control pills or drugs used to treat Parkinson's disease or psychosis.

▶ DONG QUAI

Dong quai (*Angelica sinensis*) has been used in traditional Chinese medicine for over 1,200 years to treat menstrual pain and irregularity, as well as hot flashes in menopause. Yet very little research has been conducted to test its efficacy and clinical trials to date have not shown effects on hot flashes. Caveat: Experts in Chinese medicine point out that the preparations used in these trials are not the same as those used in their practice.

Usage: Hot flashes.

Scientific proof of efficacy: Low.

Dosage: Up to 150 mg per day.

Precautions: Dong quai may interfere with blood-thinning medications, such as warfarin, heparin, or aspirin.

▶ EVENING PRIMROSE

Evening primrose oil originates from the seeds of the flowering plant *Oenothera biennis*. A rich source of omega-6 fatty acids, this oil is often recommended for treating hot flashes, although clinical trials have shown it to be no more effective than placebo. Nonetheless, combined with vitamin E, it may help with breast tenderness.

Usage: Hot flashes.

Scientific proof of efficacy: Low.

Dosage: 2–6 g per day.

Precautions: Generally well tolerated. It may increase the effects of the HIV medicine lopinavir.

▶ GINSENG AND MACA ROOT

The ginseng root is considered an adaptogenic herb, meaning it promotes resistance to external and internal stressors, thereby supporting our physical and mental health. In traditional medicine, Asian ginseng (*Panax ginseng* or *Panax quinquefolius*) and maca root (Peruvian ginseng, *Lepidium meyenii*) are said to heighten concentration, improve sexual function, and promote arousal. A systematic review of randomized controlled trials indicates that ginseng can improve symptoms of menopausal depression and low mood while supporting libido and overall well-being. Despite its success in these ways, ginseng doesn't consistently help with vasomotor symptoms, memory, or concentration.

Usage: Mood and libido.

Scientific proof of efficacy: Medium.

Dosage: 400 mg per day of standardized extract. Because of the lack of long-term safety studies, its use should be limited to a maximum of six months.

Precautions: Generally well tolerated. Insomnia is the most common side effect, so it is best taken early in the day. Other potential side effects include menstrual problems, breast pain, increased heart rate, high or low blood pressure, headache, and digestive issues. Ginseng may interfere with blood-thinning medications, such as warfarin, heparin, or aspirin.

▶ KAVA

Kava (*Piper methysticum*) is a pepper from the Pacific Islands. While kava supplements possibly reduce anxiety to some extent, they have not been shown to decrease hot flashes.

Usage: Hot flashes and anxiety.

Scientific proof of efficacy: Low.

Dosage: 50–250 mg per day.

Precautions: The FDA has issued a warning about kava because of its potential to damage the liver. Kava can also cause digestive upset, headache, and dizziness.

▶ PHYTOESTROGENS

Phytoestrogens are estrogen-like substances found in cereal, soy, vegetables, and some herbs that act as weaker estrogens in the body. The most common phytoestrogen supplements are isoflavones extracted from soy and red clover, while flaxseeds are also often recommended. A review of as many as twenty-one clinical trials indicates that phytoestrogens decrease the number and frequency of hot flashes and improve vaginal dryness. However, results differ depending on the type of phytoestrogen used, as reviewed below.

SOY ISOFLAVONES

Some soy isoflavones (such as soy protein isolate, isoflavone-rich soy extracts, or isoflavone capsules) can be effective in relieving mild-to-moderate perimenopausal hot flashes. For example, a study of 60 postmenopausal women compared soy isoflavone supplements to HRT for relief of hot flashes. After sixteen weeks, those taking isoflavones experienced a 50 percent reduction in hot flashes, while those on HRT had a 46 percent reduction. While more research is needed to confirm these results, soy isoflavones may also have positive effects on bone mineral density, reducing the risk of osteoporosis. However, they are not effective against night sweats, insomnia, or depression. Something to keep in mind is that soy effects vary according to genetic background, and only 30 to 50 percent of Western women experience beneficial effects. The main soy isoflavones are called *genistein, daidzein,* and *S-equol.*

Usage: Hot flashes.

Scientific proof of efficacy: Medium.

Dosage: 40–80 mg per day. Because of the lack of long-term safety studies, the use of isoflavones should be limited to a maximum of six months.

Precautions: Generally well tolerated. The most common side effects are gastrointestinal issues. Current evidence indicates that it's safe for women who have had or are at risk for cancer to eat soy *foods,* while it's still uncertain whether soy isoflavone supplements are safe for them. Professional societies do not endorse soy isoflavone supplements for fear of overconsumption.

RED CLOVER ISOFLAVONES

Red clover (*Trifolium pratense*) is one of the most widely researched herbs for menopausal health. According to systematic reviews, red clover isoflavones are not consistently effective for daytime hot flashes but may help relieve night sweats, especially among post-menopausal women. For example, a clinical trial of 109 postmeno-pausal women showed 80 mg of red clover isoflavones taken for ninety days reduced night sweats by an average of 73 percent.

Usage: Night sweats.

Scientific proof of efficacy: Medium.

Dosage: 80 mg per day. Red clover extracts have been used in clinical studies for as long as three years with apparent safety.

Precautions: The safety of red clover for patients with breast or endometrial cancer has not been established.

FLAXSEED

Flaxseeds, or linseeds, are good sources of lignans, a polyphenol pre-cursor to phytoestrogen activity. They also contain omega-3 fatty acids and fiber. As lignans are found in seeds' cell walls, flaxseeds must be freshly ground to release them successfully. There is no ev-idence that flaxseed helps with hot flashes, though it supports healthy digestion and may have positive effects on cholesterol.

Usage: Hot flashes.

Scientific proof of efficacy: Low.

Dosage: 25 grams (2 spoonfuls) of ground seeds daily.

Precautions: Generally well tolerated. The most common side ef-fects are digestive upsets, such as abdominal bloating, nausea, and diarrhea.

▶ RHODIOLA

Rhodiola (*Rhodiola rosea*) is an adaptogenic herb that grows in the cold high-altitude regions of Europe and Asia. Traditionally, it was used to increase endurance and avoid fatigue and burnout. Although the re-search on this herb is scant, there is some evidence that rhodiola may help balance the stress hormone cortisol while balancing blood sugar regulation. Along with regular exercise, it may help stabilize fat metab-olism during menopause and, for some women, accelerate weight-loss efforts.

Usage: Stress, fatigue, metabolic activity.

Scientific proof of efficacy: Low.

Dosage: 100 mg per day.

Precautions: Generally well tolerated over a six-to-twelve-week period. Possible side effects include dizziness and either dry mouth or excessive saliva production.

▶ ST. JOHN'S WORT

St. John's wort (*Hypericum perforatum*) is a flowering plant used in traditional European medicine as far back as the ancient Greeks. It treats anxiety, irritability, insomnia, and depression—all without affecting hormones. St. John's wort is effective for mild to moderate anxiety and depression compared to placebo, seemingly as effective as antidepressant meds (SSRIs). Based on these findings, some professional societies consider St. John's wort a viable option for short-term treatment of mild depressive symptoms and mood changes during perimenopause and after menopause.

Usage: Anxiety, mood, and depressive symptoms during perimenopause.

Scientific proof of efficacy: High.

Dosage: 900 mg per day for up to twelve weeks.

Precautions: St. John's wort can interact with various medicines and should be approached with caution. These medicines include blood thinners such as warfarin, heparin, and aspirin; digoxin (medication for heart rhythm); anticonvulsants (medications for seizures and epilepsy); antidepressant drugs (especially SSRIs or SNRIs); cyclosporin (an immune-suppressing drug); HIV medications; methadone; oral contraceptives; and some anticancer drugs.

▶ TRIBULUS

Traditionally, tribulus (*Tribulus terrestris*), also known as "herbal Viagra," has been used to energize and improve sexual function in men, but it may also be helpful for postmenopausal women. This herb contains *steroidal saponins* that, structurally similar to estrogen, may convert into weaker versions of androgens, similar to DHEA.

Usage: Low libido.

Scientific proof of efficacy: Low.

Dosage: 250–1,500 mg per day.

Precautions: Generally safe at small doses. Results are not yet in on its interactions with prescription medications; proceed with care.

▶ VALERIAN ROOT

Valerian (*Valeriana officinalis*), in the form of herbal tea or tablets, may help with insomnia and sleeplessness. Whether used on its own or in combination with lemon balm or passionflower, it can improve the sleep quality in postmenopausal women. Helpful in falling asleep and staying asleep, it may reduce nighttime waking. It may take up to four weeks of regular use to see an effect.

Usage: Sleep support.

Scientific proof of efficacy: Medium.

Dosage: The starting dose is 400 mg, one hour before bedtime. For tinctures, 2–5 droppers full.

Precautions: Generally well tolerated. It may cause headaches, dizziness, stomach upset, or fatigue for some the morning after use.

Non-Botanical Supplements

▶ B VITAMINS

B vitamins, especially vitamins B_{12} (cobalamin), B_6 (pyridoxine), B_9 (folic acid), and B_5 (pantothenic acid), are in high demand for support of cell metabolism, hormonal production, cardiovascular health, and a healthy nervous system. While there is no consistent evidence that they help reduce hot flashes, B vitamins may help reduce stress and lower the risk of osteoporosis and bone fractures.

Vitamin B_{12} is quite important for a healthy brain, especially as we get older. While our gut bacteria make a tiny amount of B_{12}, most of it must come from our diet. If you are following a strict plant-based diet without any animal foods, it's essential to supplement with vitamin B_{12} regardless of your menopausal status. If you are fifty and older, or if you suffer from gastritis, reduced stomach acid, Crohn's or celiac disease, or take medications for diabetes, acid blockers, or birth control pills, talk to your doctor about having your vitamin B status checked. All these conditions can negatively impact your B vitamin levels. If your plasma levels don't improve after three to four weeks of supplementation, you may want to try methylated B vitamins (*methylcobalamin* and *methylfolate*).

Usage: Stress and cognitive support.

Scientific proof of efficacy: Medium-high.

Dosage: For cognitive support: 500 mcg of vitamin B_{12}, 600–800 mcg of folic acid, and 10–50 mg of vitamin B_6, taken daily with food. For stress support, add 100 mg of vitamin B_5.

Precautions: Generally well tolerated. No known interactions with medications.

▶ CALCIUM AND VITAMIN D

Calcium and vitamin D are widely recommended for bone health after menopause. Ideally, calcium is best sourced from high-calcium food like spinach, cauliflower, kale, broccoli, yogurt, almonds, and canned fish with bones. You may need calcium supplements if you can't consume enough calcium with diet alone. Vitamin D helps the body absorb calcium and may improve vaginal dryness. Our primary source of vitamin D is the sun; however, for various reasons, many people are deficient in vitamin D, so supplements may help.

Usage: Bone health.

Scientific proof of efficacy: High.

Dosage: 1,200 mg of calcium from all sources (food alone or food and supplements) and 800–1,000 IU of vitamin D per day.

Precautions: Generally well tolerated. Calcium can decrease the efficacy of aspirin, levothyroxine (a thyroid medication), and some antibiotics.

▶ MAGNESIUM

Magnesium is an essential mineral that supports nerve and muscle function while playing an important role in sleep regulation. While the effects of magnesium supplements on sleep are inconsistent, many perimenopausal and postmenopausal women report relief from insomnia when using them.

Usage: Sleep support.

Scientific proof of efficacy: Low.

Dosage: Up to 3 grams of magnesium citrate one hour before bedtime. Magnesium creams are also available.

Precautions: Generally well tolerated. Magnesium can cause loose stools and diarrhea. It can decrease the efficacy of aspirin and levothyroxine (a thyroid medication).

▶ MELATONIN

A hormone produced by the brain, melatonin helps control sleep cycles. Melatonin supplements can help you fall asleep and are a common sleep aid for insomnia. If you're waking up in the middle of the night, try the extended-release preparation instead.

Usage: Sleep support.

Scientific proof of efficacy: High.

Dosage: 1–3 mg pills at bedtime for no more than two weeks. The maximum dose is 6 mg.

Precautions: Generally safe when used in the short term at recommended doses. Possible interactions with sedatives.

▶ OMEGA-3S

Omega-3 oils are anti-inflammatories that support the heart and the brain. There is emerging evidence that omega-3 supplements may help reduce night sweats and depressed mood associated with menopause. Although clinical trials are not always consistent, omega-3 supplementation has also been associated with reduced brain shrinkage, better mood, better memory, and a possibly lower risk of dementia.

Usage: Night sweats, cognitive support.

Scientific proof of efficacy: Low for night sweats; medium-high for mood and cognition.

Dosage: High-purity omega-3 fish oil or algae oil containing 500–1,000 mg DHA and 300–500 mg EPA per day.

Precautions: Moderate interactions with blood-thinning medications, such as warfarin and heparin. Too much omega-3 can result in bleeding and bruising.

▶ VITAMIN E

Vitamin E (*tocopherol*) is a fat-soluble vitamin that acts as an antioxidant in the body while also supporting the immune system. Some clinical trials report fewer hot flashes after four weeks of vitamin E supplementation. Vitamin E was also linked to a 35 to 40 percent reduction in hot flashes among breast cancer patients.

Usage: Hot flashes.

Scientific proof of efficacy: Medium-high.

Dosage: 800 IUs of a mixed tocopherol complex (containing alpha, beta, gamma, and delta tocopherols) per day.

Precautions: Moderate interactions with blood-thinning medications, such as warfarin and heparin. If you have a condition such as heart disease or diabetes, do not take more than 400 IU/day.

16

Stress Reduction and Sleep Hygiene

CLEARING THE FOG:
REDUCE STRESS, PRIORITIZE SLEEP

Our stress-inducing society celebrates productivity to a fault, seamlessly prioritizing it over sleep and rest. Laboring under the delusion that sleep can even get in the way, many of us start our professional careers or climb the ladder of success trying to prove to ourselves and the world how *little* sleep we need. It's no wonder that millions of people are living in a near-constant state of stress and sleep deprivation.

Women in particular are suffering the consequences of the times, sandwiched between unrealistic wonder-woman expectations on the one hand and our very down-to-earth roles as partners, mothers, caregivers, and active members of society on the other. As a result, women report considerably higher stress levels than men, a difference that peaks around age forty-five, when many juggle career ladders and the brunt of familial responsibilities simultaneously, discovering the "you can have it all" propaganda wasn't everything it was cracked up to be. Too many of us strain under the weight of multiplying roles, often without adequate acknowledgment, compensation, or support. This overloaded midlife moment is when we should take *extra* care of ourselves, not less. In reality, we are left with zero time to do so, between the squeeze of obligations and exhaustion.

Often, it isn't until life throws a curveball at us in the form of total burnout or any manner of illness that we are forced to readdress our relationship with sleep and inner peace. When we do, we reinstate both with the reverence they deserve, accepting that we cannot manage without them. For many women, this life lesson tends to land with menopause.

STRESS, SLEEP, AND MENOPAUSE

Stress is a little cloak-and-dagger, coming in two types, acute and chronic. Acute stress is a short-lived response to imminent danger or a high-stress event, born of the brain's instinct to protect us: there's an accident, your adrenaline skyrockets, and you slam on the brakes to avoid a crash. But the chronic stress so prevalent today is a sneakier type, sometimes low-grade but incessant. It stems from ongoing day-to-day things that happen on repeat—like commuting, getting stuck in traffic, long hours of work seated at a screen, overscheduled days, constant texting, the news, and the deadline-to-deadline pace and to-do lists of modern-day life. Slowly but surely, this *chronic* stress persistently siphons off our reserves, slowly draining our systems.

This stealth drain has become the cultural norm without our even noticing it. However, its constant drag weakens our ability to recuperate. When our bodies are taxed beyond their means for years, if not decades, there is an inevitable toll across the board—physically, emotionally, and psychologically. But what's important to realize is that chronic stress is actually bankrupting your *hormones.*

Here's how: Cortisol, our number one stress hormone, works in tandem with our sex hormones. That's because the body relies on the same molecule, called *pregnenolone,* to make both sex hormones and stress hormones, and sometimes it has to make a choice as to the lucky recipient. When you're under acute but temporary stress, your body will steal some pregnenolone away from estrogen production to make more cortisol to deal with whatever crisis. No biggie—once things calm down, your body will turn down cortisol production and resume its estrogen production as usual. There's a catch, though. When you're under *chronic* stress, your cortisol levels remain high for prolonged periods. This puts a longer-term strain on your sex hormone supply in the process, prolonging the so-called pregnenolone steal. This hormonal sleight-of-hand can in turn promote hot flashes, anxiety, and even the potential for depression. Additionally, menopause itself, depending on how you wear it, can become a chronic stressor in your life, especially when left unattended. A vicious circle of steady cortisol production and depleted sex hormones can ensue, further aggravating the symptoms of menopause, and then . . . we're really in the soup. We can find ourselves short-tempered, frazzled, or acting irrationally. We can feel empty, sluggish, and unable to gather our thoughts. Keys go missing, names escape us, and appointments are missed. And just like that, sleep is pretty much off the table, too, just when you need it most.

Once this goes on long enough, something's got to give. A growing amount of alarming science shows that chronic stress and sleep deprivation can launch a formidable attack on the body. They are major contributing circumstances in a wide range of illnesses, spanning minor conditions to the big leagues. Whether lowering your ability to recover from common colds and infections or putting you at higher risk of heart disease, cancer, and even dementia, the combo is a recipe for disaster. Case in point: Brain-imaging studies show that *for women in particular*, a high-stress life might mean memory loss and brain shrinkage by the time you hit fifty. Not getting enough time to recuperate also contributes to pain, inflammation, and an overall decreased quality of life. So while it's perfectly natural to experience stress, and sleep may be hard to come by from time to time, neither one should become the norm in your life. When the going gets tough, the tough need to *smarten up*. Let me underline that thinking clearly and feeling whole means reducing stress and prioritizing sleep. Thankfully, there are scientifically validated tools proven to work for women in particular that keep stress in check while at the same time improving restful sleep.

MIND-BODY INTERVENTIONS FOR MENOPAUSE

We have soap to clean our hands, toothpaste to brush our teeth, and shampoo to wash our hair. However, we are given no tools to cultivate our mental health. I'd argue the mind is just as essential and personal to us as any other body part, yet most of us are not raised with tools to safeguard it. Just as we want to take care of our bodies with diet, exercise, and medicine when necessary, it's time to embrace similar concepts when maintaining our minds and equilibrium.

Although many stressors cannot be eliminated, we can learn ways to keep stress in check, reduce its harmful effects on our body and mind, and even tweak how we respond to them in the first place. These coping skills are necessary to meet life's challenges and create a renewed sense of self-confidence, balance, and harmony. Simultaneously, some mind-body tools and practices promote hormonal balance, alleviating the symptoms of menopause in turn. This makes them especially handy for those interested in sidestepping pharmaceutical options. Most of all, remember that self-care is *not* selfish. *You* matter, too. Nobody can pour from an empty cup.

Yoga

Many different forms of yoga have developed and evolved across the globe since ancient times. Most practices involve physical poses or movement sequences, conscious regulation of breathing, and mindfulness techniques to increase present awareness and a sense of well-being. In several studies and clinical trials, regularly practicing yoga for at least twelve weeks positively affects the psychological symptoms of menopause, especially fatigue. Women who practice yoga also tend to have reduced symptoms of stress and insomnia, as well as an improved physical quality of life, with fewer hot flashes and urinary and vaginal issues.

Meditation and Mindfulness-Based Stress Reduction

For millennia, cultures worldwide have used meditation to cultivate physical, mental, and spiritual well-being. We have since begun to understand that this practice has the power to protect us from stress overload by modulating the activity of the brain regions in charge of worrying, thinking, and feeling.

One of the most researched relaxation techniques for menopause is mindfulness-based stress reduction (MBSR). MBSR combines a variety of exercises like mindfulness meditation, yoga, and acceptance to develop an awareness of the present moment. In a clinical trial of 110 perimenopausal and postmenopausal women, MBSR led to meaningful improvements in overall quality of life and sleep quality, as well as less stress and less anxiety. Strikingly, for some women, a combination of MBSR and cognitive therapy was just as effective at preventing depression relapse as antidepressants. You heard right—something we are capable of doing inside our minds can be as powerful as prescription medications.

Another great option is Kirtan Kriya, a chanting meditation from the Kundalini yoga tradition. Kirtan Kriya prescribes practicing the specific sounds *Saa Taa Naa Maa* accompanied by *mudras*, or hand positions, and can be done in just twelve minutes a day. Check this: The practice has been shown to reduce inflammation while improving memory, sleep, and mental clarity in as little as eight weeks. So how do you practice Kirtan Kriya? First, sit on the floor with your legs crossed or on a chair or couch. Keep the back of your neck straight and your chin slightly down. Imagine a gentle cord pulling up through the top of your head. Rest your hands on your knees with your palms facing upward. When you're ready, start chanting the sounds *Saa Taa Naa Maa*. Touch your thumb to your index finger (saying *Saa*), thumb to middle finger (*Taa*), thumb to the ring finger (*Naa*), and thumb to the pinkie finger (saying *Maa*). For a twelve-minute practice, here is the sequence:

Chant out loud for two minutes.

Chant in a whisper for two minutes.

Chant in silence for four minutes.

Chant in a whisper for two more minutes.

Chant out loud for two more minutes.

When you're done, inhale and stretch your arms up. Exhale, lower your arms, and relax for a moment. Namaste. If you prefer to practice this meditation to music, several playlists are available on Spotify, You-Tube, and other channels. If you do it on your own, try an app like Insight Timer, which lets you set intervals with gentle sounds that indicate when it's time to transition your chanting.

In summary, meditation and mindfulness training can help reduce stress, anxiety, and depressive symptoms. Just like exercise, how you meditate is a personal preference. There are many different meditation forms, techniques, and even apps available (such as Headspace or Calm), so find the one that works best for you. Then treat this like exercise: let yourself build a new kind of muscle and celebrate your success.

Hypnosis

Hypnosis is a mind-body therapy involving a deeply relaxed state of focused attention, mental imagery, and suggestion. Suggestion, in this case, refers to planting positive seeds to ease challenges or discomfort. Hypnosis has been recommended for treating menopausal symptoms by several professional societies, including the North American Menopause Society, as it can reduce hot flashes and poses little risk. In randomized clinical trials of breast cancer survivors, just five sessions of hypnotherapy resulted in a 69 percent reduction in hot flash severity and frequency.

Among women with no history of breast cancer, hypnosis also reduced hot flashes by 50 to 74 percent, which is impressive, while also improving sleep quality and sexual desire at the same time.

How can you find a specialist? Look up your country's national society of clinical hypnosis and search for a hypnotherapist that specializes in relief of menopausal symptoms or of chemotherapy-induced brain fog or other symptoms. If you live in the United States, this is the link to the website of the American Society of Clinical Hypnosis: https://www.asch.net/aws/ASCH/pt/sp/home_page.

Cognitive Behavioral Therapy (CBT)

CBT is an action-oriented psychological intervention that helps people to develop practical ways of managing problems and provides new coping skills and useful strategies. The therapy combines strategies such as education, motivational interviewing, relaxation, and paced breathing. For this reason, it can be a helpful approach because the same skills can be applied to different problems and improve well-being in general. CBT is recommended by the North American Menopause Society to treat hot flashes, as well as menopausal depression and other symptoms. Although it doesn't appear to necessarily reduce the frequency of hot flashes, it can reduce their intensity and discomfort. To find a specialist near you, you can check the websites of the main professional societies in your country for directories of certified practitioners. In the United States, for instance, details of accredited CBT therapists can be found online at the American Board of Cognitive and Behavioral Psychology's website: https://services.abct.org. If you're in the UK, you can use the CBT Register UK: www.cbtregisteruk.com.

Paced Breathing and Relaxation Training

Biofeedback, massage, and other relaxation techniques have all been used to treat menopausal symptoms. In some clinical trials, these techniques reduced the frequency of hot flashes and lessened stress and fatigue. Although these studies were not as rigorous as those regarding yoga, hypnosis, and CBT, there's no better way to see what it does for you than trying it yourself. Paced or diaphragmatic breathing, for example, is slow, even breathing that can be used to calm down your body's physical and emotional reactions. The diaphragm is located just below the lungs and forms a barrier between the lungs and the stomach. Breathing from the stomach or below the diaphragm increases lung capacity, so that we get more oxygen, which also has a significant calming effect. If practiced regularly, paced breathing can help you to relax, and may relieve hot flashes. Best results are achieved by doing this for 20 minutes, three times a day. If you feel that you don't have enough time, start by practicing this every day for 10 to 15 minutes. Immediately give it a roll when a hot flash hits, continuing for 5 minutes.

It's really easy:

> Breathe in from the belly while slowly counting to 5.
> Release the breath while slowly counting to 5.

Acupuncture

Acupuncture is a pillar of traditional Chinese medicine. Using gentle pressure or hair-fine needles, the practitioner stimulates specific points on the body that mark the body's meridians, or energy channels, to treat disease and pain. Although there is currently limited evidence that acupuncture relieves the symptoms of menopause, when performed by a highly trained practitioner, it poses a promising med-free alternative to women seeking one.

Aromatherapy

Aromatherapy, or essential oil therapy, uses naturally extracted aromatic plant essences to address various physiological and psychological imbalances. Some scented oils like lavender and verbena are believed to reduce anxiety and increase relaxation. For now, there is insufficient evidence that aromatherapy works as a stand-alone treatment for menopausal symptoms, though it may help with stress and anxiety.

OTHER THINGS THAT REDUCE STRESS

Talk It Out

The brain plays a significant role in our stress response. It does so by regulating the production of two hormones: cortisol and adrenaline. When stress strikes, cortisol and adrenaline raise your blood pressure and heart rate, which might prompt you to land a punch—or turn tail and run. That's the well-known fight-or-flight response both men and women experience when faced with danger, everyday stressors included. However, women's brains act a bit differently from men's. Research shows that as cortisol and adrenaline flood the bloodstream, women's brains release a shot of the love hormone, oxytocin, which works to be the calm amid the storm.

Scientists suspect that the release of oxytocin may be behind women's unique impulse to tend and befriend, rather than fight or flee, when under stress. This response likely evolved ages ago when our ancestors lived in hunter-gatherer communities. Given that fighting or running away is not so easy when pregnant, nursing, or caring for children and elders, women developed their own unique way of responding to danger. In such moments, they would become even more attentive to their children (tending) while putting their heads together with other women (befriending) to ensure everyone's likelihood of survival. This response speaks to our instincts to reach out to others to secure the fort when stress hits, especially in terms of bonding with other caregivers as we protect our charges.

How does this apply to menopause? When hot flashes have you tossing off layers of clothing or you can't remember what you came to the supermarket for, you're likely to feel a kinship with any woman as sweaty or forgetful as you are. You may also find solace with those who have been through menopause, having successfully navigated it through to the other side. Talking and joking with other women about the symptoms you're experiencing builds camaraderie, reassuring you that you're not alone and that those unwelcome symptoms will not last forever. Whether it's a friend, mom, mentor, or that lady at the supermarket who seems friendly, talk to them about your experiences. Not only will this give you a feeling of support, normalcy, and sisterhood, but it will also likely result in practical advice, like "Always dress in layers" and "*Never* wear synthetic underwear."

Assemble Your Support Team

Having supportive networks is a fantastic anti-stress strategy, so think of the kind of support you need to be your best self at this stage of life, as at any other. Besides some loving friends or family members to talk to, a good family doctor or ob-gyn with whom you feel comfortable discussing all the gory details is a must, as is a "menopause mentor." There are plenty of people who can easily fulfill that role. So think about what kind of support you need. Gather your crew, persevere, and prevail! Hopefully, this book will serve that purpose, too.

For those with access to networks of healthcare professionals, there are several who may be able to provide additional help. This is not necessary for everyone or all the time, but if you do need help addressing a particular problem, these can be useful resources:

- If you are feeling depressed or anxious, consider discussing your feelings with your family doctor or a mental health professional (a psychologist, therapist, or psychiatrist).
- A menopause coach or counselor who can guide you through the complexities of the transition while also providing resources, like tips on doctor referrals, yoga teachers, acupuncturists, and more.
- A physiotherapist to help with everything from joint aches to pelvic floor rehab.

- A physical trainer to help you move safely and effectively, whether it's a boxing coach to pound off any rage and frustration or a yogi to help you come back to calm.
- A nutritionist or dietitian to help you figure out a diet plan that's as yummy as it is healthy (while also referring to chapter 14 for specific foods to prioritize).

In choosing from whatever resources are available to any given person, at the end of the day, my recommendation is to invest in help and techniques that are scientifically validated, whether DIY or administered by a professional. Too often, precious time and money are squandered on random tools, supplements, or gummy bears that claim to fight menopause. While not everyone needs or has access to an array of doctors and specialists, we all can make use of tested guidance and expertise, which is what this book is about.

I Feel the Need, the Need for . . . Sleep

While society focuses on what we eat, drink, and do in our waking hours to keep healthy, the way we sleep is calling the shots more than we ever imagined. While studies waffle as to exactly how long we should sleep, reaching for those magic eight-ish hours a night is vital for the de-stressing and recharging of our minds and bodies for the day ahead. Unfortunately, our busy lives can make winding down before bed a task in and of itself. Staying asleep can also be a challenge. Finding a nighttime routine that you enjoy and is conducive to relaxation (rather than stimulation) can help you achieve better-quality sleep. Sticking to a routine will cue your body and mind to *lean into* sleep. Here are some ways to help you practice good sleep hygiene and wind down for a sweeter slumber.

▶ DIM THOSE LIGHTS

Melatonin is a natural hormone produced by the pituitary gland in the brain. When its levels increase, this hormone signals the brain that it's time to rest. Exposure to light decreases melatonin levels, giving the body mixed signals. Our bodies' evolution is based on sleeping at night and waking up with the sun, so dimming the lights *one hour or so* before bedtime can coax your brain toward restfulness. Maintaining total darkness or minimal light in the bedroom is also effective in helping you *stay* asleep. If light is unavoidable, try an eye mask.

▶ CHECK THE TEMPERATURE AND CUE THE AMBIENCE

Part of initiating sleep is a slight drop in your body temperature. If the room is too warm, your body can't lose the heat it needs to, making it more difficult to fall asleep. Keep your bedroom cool and comfortable; the sweet spot is about 67 degrees Fahrenheit or 20 degrees Celsius. These temps can also keep hot flashes at bay. Lightweight cotton pajamas are another way to support body temperature.

Creating an ambience you are drawn to for sleep is also important. Don't make your bedroom unappealing for rest! Soft lighting, comfy pillows, warm blankets, soothing colors, and a clutter-free space can transform your bedroom into a sleep sanctuary, a dedicated space to rest and unwind from the outside world. Make sure your room is quiet; and if it's not, create a background of white noise to soothe the ear. Though if a partner's flailing or snoring makes supporting an already fragile sleep impossible, earplugs can come in handy.

▶ GOOD NIGHT, PHONE

As hard as it is for everyone to part ways with phones, tablets, computers, and TVs, the blue light emitted from these devices tells your body to *stay awake*. This cue isn't just psychological; it's a physical reality. Blue light restrains the production of melatonin, your body's lullaby hormone, while increasing the production of cortisol and adrenaline instead, which are hell-bent on waking you up *and* keeping you up. At the same time, reversing these hormonal spikes disturbs your overall balance, and during menopause, this is really playing with fire. Imposing a cutoff time for your devices can signal your brain to wind down. Say good night to your phone, computer, and TV at least one hour before bed. This commitment is your pledge to put sleep back where it belongs in your healthcare lineup. If you feel that the temptation to check emails and texts might get the best of you, put your phone in flight or night mode and kiss the world good night. If you are a recovering nighttime screen user, consider taking melatonin or another sleep supplement to reacclimate, as discussed in chapter 15.

▶ KEEP THE BEAT TO A BETTER SLEEP

Your body likes relying on a rhythm when it comes to sleep. Going to bed and waking up at the same time daily gives it what it's craving. If you wake up in the middle of the night, be gentle with yourself. Keeping the lights off or dimmed, gently turn to something relaxing, like a sleep meditation, calming music, or a modulated, not-too-interesting audiobook. If using a night-light, select a soft, amber-colored one and avoid turning on any bright lights.

▶ PUT PEN TO PAPER

Do a brain dump! Writing down what's on your mind before going to bed can help you relax. Jot down a to-do list for tomorrow, note what you're grateful for, or journal about your day to clear the air for the night ahead. Once my husband brought me a tiny box of worry dolls as a souvenir. Inspired by a Mayan legend, worry dolls are small handmade dolls originating in Guatemala. There, children tell their concerns to the small dolls, one by one, before placing them under their pillow at night, less burdened. It's said that they tuck them there feeling confident that by morning, the dolls will have delivered fresh wisdom to manage the day ahead. For grown-ups, a nice notepad will do.

▶ MINDFUL MOMENTS

Another way to achieve this is to experiment with a sleep meditation to release the day's stressors. Start with just a few minutes before bed and then work your way up to fifteen or twenty minutes or longer. The best part? You don't need to take a class or even leave your home. All you need is a quiet place to sit and simmer down. If you're looking for guidance getting started, check out apps like Headspace and Calm, which make trying them a snap with free trial periods. You can find even more options on Spotify and YouTube, not to mention audio-books. Some of my favorite options are *Journey into Stillness* (audio-book) by Ramdesh Kaur, *Meditation for Beginners* by Jack Kornfield, and *Wherever You Go, There You Are* by Jon Kabat-Zinn (both available in several formats).

If meditation is not your thing, maybe music is. Like lullabies, soothing music can focus your mind on melody and rhythm while you sneak off to sleep. Some types of music even help lower your heart rate and slow your breathing. Slower tunes are ideal; those around 60 bpm do the trick. Create a playlist of your favorites to help you unwind or listen to nature sounds, like ocean waves or night crickets.

▶ AVOID SLEEP MEDS IF POSSIBLE

Over-the-counter sleep aids, benzodiazepines, and antihistamines such as diphenhydramine (Benadryl), a favorite for many women, are an ineffective solution for poor sleep. Though they might knock you out for a time, they won't be effective forever, causing other issues in the process. Before even going there, exercise your checklist—try sleep hygiene, stress reduction, exercise, diet, and supplements first. If the problem persists, certain prescription medications for menopausal symptoms, such as hormone replacement therapy or low-dose antide-pressants, can be more effective than prescription sleep meds. Also, consider seeing a sleep therapist, who can help customize the best op-tions for you.

17

Toxins and Estrogen Disrupters

HORMONE-DISRUPTING CHEMICALS

When we hear *environmental toxins,* we tend to envision nuclear plants, smoke-spewing factories, or even wildfires. The truth of the matter is more subtle than that. While such extreme short-lived instances of severe air pollution are readily identified and acted upon, so-called background levels remain constant but unmonitored, leaving millions of people susceptible to the insidious damage environmental pollution can cause.

Toxic substances enter the atmosphere—and consequently the very air we breathe—from all sorts of places. While gas emissions from industrial sources like vehicle exhaust, heating units, industrial machinery, power plants, combustion engines, and cars are well-known health hazards, most toxins hit much closer to home and are unwittingly absorbed through our household products, cosmetics, and even food. These toxins can be found almost anywhere, probably more so than you may imagine. They are in the plastics used to store food, water, and a multitude of ingestible and absorbable products. They are in herbicides, pesticides, and hormonal preparations to grow our foods. We find them in our water supply due to contamination from agriculture and manufacturing, and there are flame retardants in clothes, cars, toys, and home furnishings.

In the last seventy years, nearly 100,000 new chemicals have been released into the environment via our food and water supply. At least 85 percent of these chemicals have never been tested for their health effects in humans, so their safety quotient is unknown. Among those that have been tested, as many as 800 chemicals are either known or suspected to negatively impact our health, especially our hormones.

These substances are called endocrine-disrupting chemicals (EDCs), or hormone disrupters. They do precisely what the name implies: they seriously mess with your hormones. EDCs are chemical contaminants that mimic your natural hormones and, in doing so, sneak in and scramble the messages your cells are meaning to communicate to one another. Many EDCs mimic estrogen in particular, and are known as xenoestrogens, or foreign estrogens. Think of them as estrogen's evil twin. By sending mixed messages to estrogen receptors, they trigger hormonal imbalances throughout the reproductive system, which have been linked to premature puberty, miscarriages, infertility, endometriosis—even some cancers. Worse, because they're very easily absorbed, xenoestrogens enter your body at much higher concentrations than your own estrogen, damaging the function of the endocrine system while harming the nervous system as well. It hurts to put too fine a point on this, but hundreds of these chemicals are also toxic to *your brain*. Just in recent years, air pollution alone has become both an acknowledged health hazard and a newly identified risk factor for stroke and dementia! Similar concerns have been raised about many other chemical toxins.

While rigorous research on this topic is still ongoing, this is what we know so far:

- It only takes small amounts of hormone-disrupting chemicals to damage our health. Even low-level exposure to xenoestrogens can do significant toxic harm to children and women—especially pregnant women. Many babies are born already carrying a toxic load of hundreds of environmental chemicals in their bodies. The American Academy of Pediatrics recommends limiting exposure to environmental pollutants and chemicals—plastic in particular—for infants and children.

- Hormone-disrupting chemicals are stored in our body fat. Since women are built with more fat tissue than men, we accumulate these toxins at even higher levels. The highest concentration can be found in breast tissue, which correlates with an increased risk of breast cancer.

- The accumulated effect of these toxins can last for years, if not for life.

- Many manufactured chemicals remain in the environment for decades. DDT, for example, a pesticide banned in the United States in 1972, can still be found in the soil to this day. We also find it in the bloodstream of people born long after all usage ceased. Another excellent example of a chemical substance that can last hundreds of years is one we're all aware of by now: plastic.

- Pollutants concentrate in living organisms through bio-accumulation. That means their levels build up in your body every time you are exposed. We're not the only ones in this boat. Animals carry toxins in their bodies, too. This is especially concerning in the case of farm animals, since whatever toxins they store end up contaminating the meat and dairy products we eat.

Overall, we are constantly exposed to thousands of substances that can wreak havoc on our hormones. The primary culprits are:

- *Cigarette smoke.* It contains not only nicotine but also arsenic, 1,3-butadiene, and carbon monoxide, as well as additional nitrosamines, aldehydes, and other chemicals that increase the risk of various cancers.

- *Bisphenol A (BPA).* Found in plastics such as water bottles, plastic containers, thermal liners, the inner lining of canned foods, plastic utensils, and cups.
- *Phthalates.* Found in soft plastics such as vinyl flooring, shower curtains, food packaging, children's lunch boxes, toys, and teethers, as well as fragrances and body care products.
- *PFOA and PTFE.* Found in the linings and coatings of much of our cookware, released when heated.
- *Brominated and organophosphate flame retardants.* Found in rugs, foam furniture, carpets, floor polish, nail polish, clothing, and other textiles.
- *Insecticides/pesticides.* Found in bug sprays, termite control, lawn and garden treatments, and animal flea and tick control treatments.

WAYS TO REDUCE ENVIRONMENTAL POLLUTANTS IN YOUR LIFE

As individuals, we can't always control or eliminate all of our exposure to toxins. Nor can we single-handedly fix the policies around environmental health. Nonetheless, the change begins with us—how we live our lives and raise our children. While the weight of this responsibility can be intimidating, cutting down such a tall order into chunks can help. If we step back and make small choices each day in an ecologically health-conscious way, we might find that progress is possible. While some options can be expensive, like electric cars and solar panels, many others aren't.

By All Means, Quit Smoking

Despite consciousness-raising around cigarette-related cancers, lung disease, and heart disease, smoking remains an ongoing public health issue worldwide. In the United States alone, more people die from smoking cigarettes than from HIV, illegal drug use, alcohol use, car crashes, and guns *combined*. Still today, approximately 20 percent or nearly 60 million Americans smoke. A remarkable 88 million non-smokers, including children, are exposed to secondhand and third-hand smoke every year.

The list of negatives attached to smoking cigarettes is a long one. Still, most people don't realize that in addition to their well-known risks, cigarettes have profoundly adverse effects on our hormones. In fact, no lifestyle factor single-handedly does more damage to your ovaries than smoking. Consider this: Young women who smoke have a significantly higher risk of painful menstrual cycles and infertility than nonsmokers. That's in part because nicotine stifles your body's ability to turn testosterone into estrogen, making it harder for your ovaries to supply you with estrogen. As a result, smoking makes hormonal symptoms even *worse* than they have to be. As we go through menopause, cigarette smoking then amplifies the symptoms everyone's trying to avoid. Hot flashes, anxiety, mood swings, and insomnia are all the more intense and frequent for women who smoke than for those who don't.

Additionally, by making your estrogen levels fall faster, smoking brings on menopause *sooner*. Women who smoke 100 cigarettes (5 packs) *in their entire lives* have a 26 percent greater risk of going through menopause in their forties as compared to nonsmokers. So we're looking at a habit that can kick-start early menopause while simultaneously intensifying its symptoms, depriving you of the beneficial effects of estrogen in the process. This bet is a lose-lose gamble if ever there was one. If that weren't enough, smoking stokes the risk of heart disease for women on HRT.

Unfortunately, if you're a nonsmoker frequently exposed to others' smoke, all the risks discussed above apply to you, too. Keeping clear of cigarette smoke and encouraging others to quit smoking around you is all the more important to safeguarding everyone involved. As some important incentives, quitting smoking and reducing exposure to passive smoke can dramatically improve a person's overall health, uplift mood, increase energy, and improve sleep. This trade-off is hard to beat.

According to many healthcare professionals, quitting for good may require a combination of behavioral and pharmacologic therapies. Nicotine replacement therapy (NRT), cognitive behavioral therapy (the CBT we reviewed in the previous chapter), antidepressants with anxiety-relieving properties, exercise, and acupuncture can all be helpful. The American Cancer Society, the American Lung Association, and the National Cancer Institute all provide online resources and chat support. Also keep in mind that a healthful diet rich in antioxidants (with a little help from vitamin C and E supplementation if needed) is truly important for smokers, ex-smokers, and those exposed to passive smoke.

Filter Indoor Air

An indoor air purifier is always a worthy investment, especially if you are exposed to cigarette smoke at home or live in a high-traffic area or industrial zone. Also, between the volume of toxins in home-building materials, furnishings, and electronics and the hundreds of chemicals hiding in household cleaners, insecticides, body products, and cosmetics, the air *inside* your home may be just as polluted as the air *outside* it.

Bringing potted plants into your home can also help to minimize indoor pollution. Several common plants reduce volatile organic compounds (VOCs), like formaldehyde, xylene, toluene, benzene, chloroform, ammonia, and acetone, all commonly found in many homes. These natural helpers include snake plants, spider plants, peace lilies, and golden pothos, to name a few.

Use Eco-Friendly Household Products

Our home cleaning products leave residue along all surfaces, settle into our bedding and upholstery, and imbue the air we breathe. We ingest, inhale, and absorb these chemicals throughout our day. While eco-friendly household cleaning products can be more expensive, even traditional supermarket chains now carry them. Once-exclusive labels like Mrs. Meyer's and Seventh Generation can now be found at accessible prices in places like Costco, Target, and your local supermarket. It's also possible to mix your own cleaning products, a less expensive solution than store-bought. It's impressive what vinegar and baking soda can do!

Green Up Your Home

Fabric protectant chemicals and flame retardants are two classes of seriously harmful endocrine disrupters built into your sofas, chairs, carpeting, and other household decor. Minimize exposure by emphasizing wood, metals, untreated natural fibers, and other eco-friendly upholstery. Just as important, dress for health. Some flame retardants present in many clothes and pajamas, especially those containing synthetic fibers, are known endocrine disrupters. Instead, select cotton and untreated natural fibers as much as possible. Among other things, they are recommended for women experiencing hot flashes, as synthetic fabrics make you sweat more.

Clean Food and Water

Given that most people eat at least three times a day, every day, paying attention to our food choices is an integral part of avoiding contaminants. More than 14,000 hormone-disrupting chemicals are found in our food supply alone. By far, ultra-processed food is the premier source of our chemical overload, given the high quantity of additives, thickeners, emulsifiers, and synthetic preservatives lurking in these products to enhance flavor, appearance, or texture or to extend their shelf life.

Additionally, as many as 25 percent of the pesticides routinely sprayed on fruit and vegetables are known to disrupt estrogen levels—not to mention the many others we've yet to test. Dairy and meat products from commercially raised animals are also likely to contain contaminants, given that all sorts of chemicals are routinely mixed into the animals' feed to make them grow larger, faster.

If you are not sure whether a food is safe to consume, here are two fundamental rules:

▶ CHECK THE INGREDIENTS LABEL

The most common and worst-for-you food additives are high-fructose corn syrup, hydrogenated and partially hydrogenated fats, monosodium glutamate (MSG), artificial food coloring (for example, Blue 1, Red 3, Red 40, Yellow 5, and Yellow 6), sodium nitrate, gums (guar and xanthan gum), carrageenan, and sodium benzoate. Do your level best to avoid ingesting these. Preservatives that are actually safe to consume include ascorbic acid (vitamin C), citric acid, vitamin E (tocopherol), and calcium phosphate.

▶ WHEN YOU CAN, SHOP ORGANICALLY AND LOCAL

Eating organic prevents exposure to pesticides, herbicides, antibiotics, and a myriad of other chemicals in your local food supply while also preventing exposure to chemicals from other countries through imported produce and meats. Organic crops are generally grown without synthetic pesticides, artificial fertilizers, or irradiation (a form of radiation used to kill bacteria). Animals grown on organic feed are raised without antibiotics or synthetic growth hormones.

I know that choosing to buy organic food isn't always possible due to financial and access restrictions. We can only do our best, and yes, it is unfair that healthy food is more expensive than less healthy choices. However, not all foods need to be organic. When making the call on when to buy organic and when to buy conventional, the Environmental Working Group (EWG) provides up-to-date information on which foods contain the most pesticides. Currently, the Dirty Dozen (the EWG's list of products vulnerable to contamination) includes apples, celery, berries, peaches, spinach, and kale, so these are the ones you might want to invest in by buying organic. The Clean Fifteen, produce like avocados, cabbage, corn, and pineapples, are the least affected, so you can skip buying their organic versions. For the rest, rinsing your vegetables and fruit will dilute the pesticides present. Peeling also helps.

If you eat animal foods, another place you want to go organic is with meat and dairy. The most contaminated products come from beef and lamb, as well as dairy milk. Chicken, turkey, and duck are safer to consume. If you eat fish, make sure it's low-mercury. Examples include anchovies, Atlantic mackerel, catfish, clams, crab, flounder, haddock, mullet, pollock, and salmon. While there are no government-approved organic standards for seafood, wild-caught fish is healthier and safer than farm-raised fish. Frozen or canned wild-caught fish is cheaper than fresh fish and just as nutritious.

Glass Is the New Plastic

Reducing the number of endocrine disrupters you absorb from plastic daily is vital for hormone balance. Getting the plastic out of your life, especially from your food sources, is officially essential. Easy hacks for eliminating much of the plastic in your fridge and pantry can be accomplished with these simple swaps:

- Use glass or stainless-steel storage containers and glass jars. Being selective this way is a good investment because you keep reusing these containers repeatedly. Affordable containers are readily available at places like Walmart or Target or online at Amazon.
- Swap out your water bottles, too. Instead of drinking out of plastic or Styrofoam, opt for glass or stainless steel. Simply reusing a glass water bottle is an affordable and cheap way to replace plastic. More and more cafés are happy to serve you using your ecological BYOC!
- Ditch nonstick pots and pans and use cast iron, stainless steel, tempered glass, or enamel instead.

- Avoid foods that come in soft plastic wrap (for example, cheese and cold cuts) or those stored in plastic.
- *Never heat food up in plastic*—even those sold to do so. BPA and other microplastics leach directly into your food whenever you microwave or reheat food in plastic containers.
- Avoid hot takeout in plastic containers. A work-around is to order cold food, like sushi. If you order hot food, remove it from those containers immediately.
- When you can, order or shop for foods in bulk and use your own cloth bags for both shopping and storing.
- Opt for reusable or refillable household products (everything from dish soap to skincare) that come in either recycled or glass containers. Then use glass jar dispensers and buy less expensive refill versions to fill them.

Be Choosy About Your Personal Care Products

Most commercial personal care products and cosmetics are laden with toxic ingredients. The same goes for body products ranging from shampoos and deodorants to sunscreens and moisturizers. Learn to read labels, and avoid ingredients known to be especially harmful. If you're unsure, visit EWG Skin Deep (www.ewg.org/skindeep) or Campaign for Safe Cosmetics (www.safecosmetics.org) for more information on companies that use clean ingredients and have eco-friendly policies. Many apps are also available to make research a snap, with product safety scores to shortcut the small print.

If upgrading your personal care products feels overwhelming, start by swapping out those items that cover the largest skin surface, like your body wash and moisturizer. Your skin absorbs up to 60 percent of what you put on it, which ends up in your bloodstream, so it makes sense to take care of these items first. The "clean beauty" movement is more mainstream every day, and the choices are endless. And there are plenty of DIY options, too. For example, try using coconut oil to remove your makeup at night. Just massage a few drops over your eyes, face, and lips; rub it off with a soft cloth; and you're done. It's magic!

In the end, eliminating many pollutants from your life isn't as hard as it may at first sound. By paying more attention to your everyday choices, you will not only dramatically decontaminate your environment and that of your loved ones but also do your part to lighten the carbon footprint on our beautiful planet. Remember, we're in this for the long haul.

18

The Power of a Positive Mindset

RETHINKING MENOPAUSE

When my husband turned forty, Facebook greeted him with an ad to buy a shiny new car. When it was my turn, I opened my messages to an ad for Botox instead.

As a society, we are led to think that when men age, they do so like a fine wine. As if they were a treasured vintage, the older they get, the more they appreciate in value. What a lovely way to embrace aging, right? However, please mind the gap. When women age, the viewpoint shifts. Age doesn't increase our appeal; instead, our maturing wine is often viewed as . . . vinegar. Social mores, both current and classic, reveal the sting of a double standard when it comes to gender and aging. For women, there seems to be a cultural expiration date after which our value falls. We have been made to believe that once we reach midlife, we've passed our peak. When viewed objectively, this directive is tough to take seriously, particularly compared to the enthusiastic greenlighting men receive at the same time. Yet the messaging is ever present, woven into marketing campaigns, coloring our cultural rhetoric in ways subtle and not.

This double standard is more apparent than ever in the myth of menopause. Historically, menopause has been treated as a pre-death condition, a pivot from which women turn toward the status of crone. Our worth and femininity have been selectively tied up in our reproductive capacity by narrow and often misogynistic standards. Not so long ago, the message of our male-dominated society would have been a curt "over and out" as we arrived at this gateway. We have been made to feel that nobody wants to hear our story; some of us might even be convinced that this is a story too embarrassing to tell. At the same time, menopause is understood as a deficiency, a syndrome dominated by symptoms, their cures, and an overall loss of well-being. The medical language of menopause is a reflection of that bias. As Dr. Jen Gunter, a fierce women's health advocate, aptly stated in *The Menopause Manifesto*: "It's common to say that the ovarian supply of eggs has been exhausted, but the concept of failure or fatigue is never applied to the penis."

Women are often measured by things we cannot and should not be expected to control—whether it's our age, every inch of our silhouette, or our menstruation status. But none of those measurements will ever reflect who you are or what you're made of. Your experiences, thoughts, actions, and accomplishments are the only worthy indicators of what's inside your mind and heart. And the only metric that's worth remembering about midlife is that it is precisely what the term implies: *the middle*. If this phase of life starts with a deep respect for what your brain and body can achieve *and have achieved*, then you are poised to usher in the kickoff of even richer and more fulfilling seasons ahead.

I hope the past chapters armed you with an understanding of how your body and brain change in midlife and during menopause, and an appreciation for the intelligent adaptations they make in the process. Understanding what menopause is and isn't, and that many solutions are available, can make the transition less uncomfortable, if not sanctioned for empowerment instead. In fact, menopause is an excellent time to shape a new chapter of your life and create a healthy, meaningful, and vibrant You.2.0. What tips the scales? Your mindset.

Konenki

As soon as we hit menopause, Western women are chided by a deafening chorus of U's: unattractive, unhappy, useless, and so on. The message here is loud and clear, and it comes at us from all directions—television, advertising, people at work, even friends who are dealing with the same challenges: *Menopausal women: You have served your purpose. Now please clear the deck.*

The impulse to quickly deal with the problem comes across even in the language we use. In English, *menopause* boils down to "monthly stop," referring to, in this case, menstruation ceasing. This in and of itself gives no greater meaning to this life stage than the fact that our period stops. And then you're on your own.

What I find particularly striking is the complete absence of any sense of achievement or gain in status associated with becoming menopausal. On the contrary, many societies in both the East and the West experience this milestone as a kickoff of a new phase of women's lives—one that can even move you to a place of honor. Interestingly, in societies where age is more revered and the older woman is considered wiser and superior, women report significantly fewer bothersome symptoms, too.* The uptick in cultural status also corresponds to an easier time going through menopause across the globe.

For instance, the Japanese word for menopause is *konenki*. Literally translated, *ko* means renewal and regeneration, *nen* means year or years, and *ki* means season or energy. The Japanese define the same event we dread—menopause—as a much lengthier and spiritual transition where the end of periods is just one element. It is telling, then, that only about 25 percent of Japanese women reportedly experience hot flashes, a considerably lower rate than in the United States. Chilliness, ironically enough, is a more common symptom, though shoulder

---

* Disclaimer: These findings are not intended to be generalized to all women of the cultures mentioned; there is of course considerable diversity within these populations.

stiffness and frozen shoulders are by far the most bothersome among Japanese women.

Similarly, some communities in India associate the experience of menopause with freedom and liberation—and their most common complaint is not hot flashes but a decrease in vision. In some Islamic, African, and Indigenous societies, menopause is also celebrated as a welcome transition; women no longer have to observe strict gender roles and may enjoy greater social freedom. Postmenopausal women actually gain status and often serve as community leaders. For another example, rural Mayan women, who also gain in social status after menopause, do not report *any* symptoms. That's although they tend to go through menopause quite early, at around age forty-four, and their estrogen levels drop just like any other woman's. Last, Native American women do not have a single word for menopause and regard the transition as a neutral or positive experience. In what is the most fitting metaphor I've come across, they describe menopause as simply "a process of ageing, like a ring around a tree."

It may be that women in other cultures are not encouraged to express their discomfort as we are in Western countries, or that lifestyle, diet, and climate protect them against menopause—or it may be that our minds have much more power over our bodies than we realize. It's probably all of the above and then some. While the biological explanations for menopausal symptoms are certainly valid, there's more to menopause than just the action of our hormones. Knowing that hot flashes and other symptoms are not mandatory shows us that we *do* have a lot more control over our own experience of menopause than we might have thought. Perhaps the greatest news is that if we choose to, we can benefit from modern medicine when needed, while at the same time seeing menopause through the eyes of different cultures: as a profoundly useful and spiritual time.

Mind Over Menopause

Numerous studies have demonstrated that a positive outlook on life in general, including embracing the aging process, is a strong predictor of physical health and emotional well-being in old age. This underscores the influential role our expectations and beliefs play in shaping our actual outcomes, regardless of the genetics and biology we have been dealt. Defying the negative stereotypes that surround menopause can be just as satisfying a pursuit, challenging societal norms and embracing the transformative power of this life stage. The experience of menopause is tied to more than what's happening within our bodies. Our own attitudes as well as the perspectives of friends, family, and society at large all color our experiences. Our inner language matters, too. Many women do not have an inherent fear of menopause but rather of what it signifies. We didn't write this story, yet we're expected to live it. And live it, we do.

Research shows a direct two-way link between a woman's physical symptoms, her beliefs about menopause, and her actual experience of the transition. For example, women who experience disruptive symptoms such as frequent and severe hot flashes tend to have more negative attitudes, which is understandable. But the reverse is also true. Women who harbor more apprehension about menopause ahead of the fact tend to experience worse symptoms throughout it. When we view menopause as a disease, we perceive this period of our lives as a "sick" time, a time when we are patients waiting for recovery.

On the other hand, women who hold positive attitudes toward menopause often report milder symptoms and a smoother transition. Also worth considering is data showing that two women reporting the same exact number of hot flashes might also report very different levels of distress regarding those symptoms. While one person may find them extremely stressful, another may simply brush them off. This discrepancy could be due to variations in psychological or emotional well-being. For example, women with better overall health, effective coping mechanisms, or a stronger support system tend to exhibit greater resilience in response to menopausal symptoms. This further demonstrates that mindset and support matter. In fact, those who report having embraced, rather than resisted, their menopause—and more broadly the aging process—often find themselves more comfortable and confident in their own skin than ever before.

You Are What You *Think*

We each see life through our own unique lens. This lens is forged of all our assumptions and expectations about ourselves, our life, and the situations around us. Our perspectives impact our perceptions of reality—influencing how we think, feel, and even physiologically respond. An intriguing example of this is a scientific phenomenon known as the *placebo effect*. This well-known factor reveals that if someone is convinced they will feel better after taking a particular medicine, they often do, even if the medicine is inactive. In fact, research shows that as many as 30 to 40 percent of people in clinical trials can experience significant improvement in their symptoms simply by taking a placebo (a sugar pill), if they believe it will help them.

So far, so good. But now consider the *nocebo effect*. This is the opposite of the placebo effect, referring to a person's negative expectations about a medicine or its potential side effects. In clinical trials, if participants are unaware they are receiving a placebo and believe they may experience harmful effects, they may indeed develop adverse side effects in response to that inert sugar pill. All of this is an excellent barometer of how powerful our minds are: what we anticipate affects our experience.

How do we apply this framework to menopause? Well, if you fear the experience will be catastrophic or can victimize you, you may notice your symptoms more, feel them more severely, or even experience less relief from therapeutic benefits. On the contrary, if you believe menopause is just a phase and that you'll be fine, even through its twists and turns, you might have a much better menopause than you would otherwise. Mindset matters. Paying attention to our belief systems pays off. Put them under the microscope. Be curious about their origin, ascertain whether their message is valid, and observe how they impact you. Being wise about whether they're supportive of your needs or setting you up for failure can be decisive. Most important, we can change our entire philosophy about menopause by becoming aware that many beliefs are not universal truths. Try to catch yourself before you retreat into negative habits. You can anticipate menopause as a shutting down or see it as an opening up. Whichever you choose, it's yours to experience.

DEVELOPING A POSITIVE MINDSET: A HOW-TO

The entire field of cognitive therapy is based on the idea that your thoughts influence your feelings—and that you can modify negative thoughts and beliefs with practice and persistence. Every thought you have affects how you feel and how you perceive your reality, and you're the one who has the last word as to what you think in the first place. No matter society's suggestions, family labels, or history itself, you and you alone have the ultimate power to pick and choose your thoughts and, in doing so, shift your reality.

We are all faced with different challenges in our day-to-day lives, many of which we may not be able to change. However, it's *how* we approach and play the hand dealt to us that can make all the difference. Having the presence of mind to do this is not necessarily easy, but opening our perspectives and being intentional about it is essential. By understanding, adapting, and shifting our mindsets, we can improve our health, decrease stress, and become more resilient to life's challenges—menopause included.

Mind Your Self-Talk

All day long, your mind carries on a running internal dialogue. If you take a moment to eavesdrop on this interior conversation, you may be surprised at its tone and content. Have you ever caught yourself mentally rehearsing the worst possible outcome of any given situation, telling yourself you can't or shouldn't do something or worrying about what you already did? Add all that to the moments you may be in the middle of a hot flash or functioning on compromised sleep, and that little voice in your head becomes *really* strident. What do you hear it say? Is it encouraging you or shooting you down? Does it support you through the difficulty—or criticize you for not being stronger, better, or above it all?

Getting a handle on our self-talk is one of the hardest things many of us will ever attempt, yet is one of the most important. The therapeutic effects of positive self-talk on our attention and emotional regulation are so well established that developing this skill is not only the core curriculum for performance enhancement programs in sports but the heart of most psychological and mindfulness-based therapies. CBT, narrative psychology, and neuroscience all agree that we can improve our self-talk by becoming conscious of undermining attitudes and beliefs. Once you've identified these, seeking evidence of more positive (and sometimes more accurate) counter stories can actively rescript self-talk in a more productive direction. Here are some of the top steps to develop positive self-talk:

- *Choose a mantra or affirmation.* In sports, one way to create more positive self-talk is to choose a mantra you can use in challenging situations. The mantra could be a simple affirmation, such as "I can do this," or a guiding suggestion, like "Breathe in, breathe out." Any simple, positive phrase you can embrace and easily remember can be a way of setting a new course, especially amid challenging moments.
- *Practice multiple scenarios.* Once you have developed the habit of repeating this phrase to the point that it's automatic, start expanding the dialogue so that you have familiar and comfortable affirmations for various situations. For example,

if you are having a hot flash, you might say, "I know the drill; I've got this." Or "Keep on going; this, too, shall pass." Or practice the deep belly breathing we reviewed in chapter 16.

- *Speak to yourself in the third person.* Sometimes we all need a good pep talk. Who better to receive that motivation from than yourself? One can imagine this kind of coaching in singles tennis, for example, which, not unlike menopause, can sometimes feel like a solitary endeavor. When you're going through a trying time, take a step back and talk to yourself as if you were your own trainer. "Come on, I believe in you," or "Take a deep breath, I'm in your corner."
- *Practice loving-kindness.* We all get impatient with our bodies from time to time, blaming them for their tribulations; for getting sick, for feeling unwell, or not changing fast enough. When you feel frustrated or nervous, pretend your body is a small child or a dear friend—anyone needing help. Tap into your impulse to extend love and support. Remember, *your body loves you.* Every cell in your entire body is working tirelessly day after day so that you may thrive. Be thankful for all it has done for you over the years, and give back when it needs you most.

Don't Worry About Fixing Yourself

Despite the rhetoric, you aren't broken. Menopause is an inevitable facet of a woman's life. While the symptoms are no fun, the journey is less bumpy now that we have choices for therapies and lifestyle interventions. If you are interested in taking medications or trying out CBT, speak to your doctor about the best options for you. At the same time, keep in mind that you're also allowed to trust the hammock of biology, letting your body work this out and depending on it to do its thing.

Laugh It Up

As the old saying goes, laughter is the best medicine. As simple as it sounds, the physical act of laughing, even without humor, is linked to complex chemical bonuses in the body that can reduce stress and increase pain tolerance. Laughter is a potent endorphin releaser, activating the neurotransmitter serotonin, your body's native antidepressant. It also has anti-inflammatory effects that help protect the heart.

Keep a Journal of Your Experience

Write your own user's manual. You're the expert on *you*. If you have a symptom bugging you, consider tracking it to notice any patterns. For example, you may discover that when you drink coffee, your sleep suffers, or that every time you watch the news, a hot flash sneaks up on you. Get to know your body's natural rhythms and reactions by nonjudgmentally observing and recording what surfaces. Track the clues and find relief.

Use Your Emotions as Tools

Like puberty, menopause is a time of intense hormonal flux and the corresponding emotional and physical changes accompanying it. Unlike your fifteen-year-old self, though, you are now an adult, able to metabolize the feelings that come up (instead of their "metabolizing" you). When sadness comes up, you may glimpse an opportunity to acknowledge or let go of something. When anger arises, it might provide an inkling as to what is asking for your protection, boundaries, or advocacy. Should fear surface, see where you may need reassurance or support. Use your emotions to learn more about yourself and better guide your choices.

Gratitude Is Not a Platitude

Although we practice looking at the glass half full rather than half empty, it's important to remember that the glass is also *refillable*. A great way to hone a bulletproof mindset is to keep track of what's good around us, otherwise known as a gratitude journal. I started keeping a family gratitude journal, and every day at dinnertime, we all come up with one to three things for which we're grateful. The idea is to cite a good event, experience, or person in your life and to sit in the positive emotions that come along with this. I find it refills our glasses. Here are some tips to get you started:

- *Be specific.* "I'm grateful that my husband brought me soup when I wasn't feeling well yesterday" will be more effective than "I'm grateful for soup."
- *Go for depth over breadth.* Elaborating in detail about a particular person or thing for which you're grateful carries more weight than a quick inventory of multiple items.
- *Get personal.* Focusing on people for whom you are grateful hits home harder than counting those things you appreciate.
- *Try subtraction, not just addition.* Consider your life *without* certain people or things rather than just tallying up all the good stuff. Be grateful for the unfavorable outcomes you avoided or turned into something positive—try not to take that good fortune for granted.
- *See good things as gifts.* Thinking of the good things in your life as gifts guards against taking them for granted. Relish and savor the gifts you've received.
- *Cherish surprises.* Try to record unexpected or surprising events, as these tend to elicit even purer pops of gratitude.

PERENNIAL OR ANNUAL?

Middle age is an obsolete term—one that should be retired, and with good reason. Traditionally, being a middle-aged or, worse still, menopausal woman implied that you've reached a cutoff date after which you can expect a swift decline. Western society wants to reassure you that you needn't worry—nobody's watching. In fact, you're promised full invisibility from now on. Deemed irrelevant by a society that worships youth in lieu of wisdom or experience, you are supposed to fade into the sunset. In many civilizations, the menopausal woman has been shown the proverbial door.

It is up to us to dump this pathetic anachronistic rhetoric. We needn't buy into archaic social norms designed to mandate when we should be done with our lives and what we are worth. Aging is not what it once was. Although getting older is an inevitable fact of life, how we age is fast evolving, no longer the arbiter of who we are and how we behave. Being older doesn't equate with feeling old any longer, or with fragility or weakness. Most women are clear that being in our forties or fifties or any other decade has nothing to do with letting ourselves go. We're not all in crisis, nor are we necessarily interested in retreating into a quiet, behind-the-scenes existence, knitting or baking pies. We have the courage and confidence to follow our passions and pursue our next moves bravely, regardless of our assigned age. What we choose to do is *our* business, and up to us.

When I heard the term *perennial* used as an alternative to *middle-aged* or *older,* I was sold. The word literally means indefinite or everlasting, and is perfectly suited to describe the new generation of ever-blooming, entirely relevant people functioning independently of their age markers. Perennials live in the present day, knowing what's happening in the world and engaging with a variety of people, peers and otherwise. Being perennial is about staying curious, creative, and passionate about taking risks, even when the world tells you otherwise.

Nobody puts a perennial in the corner.

I don't know about you, but I'll take the plus of being a perennial over the old idea I'm an annual any day. What we ultimately achieve in our perennial years is no less important than what we've achieved before then. Given what we've pulled off already, this is saying a lot. Upgrading our mindsets to live our best lives no matter our point in time will not only impact our own happiness and fulfillment but also provide a role model for our daughters and the world around them.

For this to occur, we must say no to gender ageism, and with that refusal, free menopause from its predefined state of resignation. Thanks, but no thanks—we shall not uncomfortably fade into old age. Fundamentally, it's time to rid ourselves of the stigma surrounding this stage of life, the attempt to quash half of humanity.

Let's imagine a society where the fact that you are a menopausal woman is not overlooked or ignored but noticed, valued, and lauded. Imagine a culture that allows women to embrace their various metamorphoses in peace and respect. Despite old edicts to the contrary, we are a collective, communal force with which to be reckoned. As we close this chapter, we do so aligned with a better tomorrow, a time in which there is a growing body of reliable information, as well as tailor-made healthcare, for women of all ages. It is my hope that the discussion of menopause both within the ivory towers of science and among women over coffee will continue, and that women across all cultures will find ways to embrace and find meaning and purpose in this transition—as we each add one more well-deserved ring to our tree of life.

In closing, let's circle back to the very question that marked the beginning of this book. Are you losing your mind during menopause? No, you're *getting a brand-new one.*

ACKNOWLEDGMENTS

TO ALL THE INDIVIDUALS and collectives whose input and support brought this book to life, I extend my deepest gratitude.

Caroline Sutton, my editor at Avery/Penguin Random House, along with her exceptional team of assistants, copyeditors, designers, and publicists, particularly Anne Kosmoski and Farin Schlussel—your guidance and expertise have been invaluable.

I am once again most thankful to Katinka Matson, my literary agent, for endorsing my vision and guiding it into fruition.

Sincere appreciation goes to my team at the Women's Brain Initiative and Alzheimer's Prevention Program at Weill Cornell Medicine/NewYork-Presbyterian. Without all of you, the research integral to this book wouldn't have been possible. Special thanks to our chairman, Dr. Matthew E. Fink, for giving me the opportunity to start the program in the first place, and to our many internal and external collaborators. For some honorable mentions, Schantel Williams, Drs. Susan Loeb-Zeitlin and Yelena Havryulik, the ob-gyn department, the Biomedical Imaging Center, and the department of biostatistics at Weill Cornell; and Dr. Alberto Pupi and Valentina Berti at the department of nuclear medicine of the University of Florence, Italy. Our research would not have been possible without the generous funding from the National Institute of Health/National Institute on Aging, Maria Shriver's Women's Alzheimer's Movement, the Cure Alzheimer's Fund, and the many benefactors who have blessed us with philanthropic support to our program.

My wholehearted gratitude goes to my friend and mentor, Dr. Roberta Diaz Brinton, a true trailblazer in the field of menopause. Her wisdom, knowledge, and support have been endless throughout my career.

I am deeply grateful to Maria Shriver, whose unwavering brilliance and advocacy have been invaluable to our work and continue to motivate us to do more and better. Her second foreword for my book is indeed a double blessing. Profound thanks to the ever-supportive Sandy Gleysteen on Maria's team, whose enthusiasm and efficiency are a testament to her exceptional character.

A huge thanks to the many friends and colleagues worldwide who continuously inspire me with their knowledge, experience, and passionate support of women's health. Your perspectives have been invaluable in shaping the book's ideas. To all the women and individuals who are standing up for their peers, challenging societal norms, and helping to dismantle the taboos surrounding menopause and women's brain health—your courage and efforts are creating a world where all stages of a woman's life are celebrated and understood.

I thank Veronica Wasson, Jessi Hempel, Evan Hempel, and Kyle for their feedback and insights. Your sensitivity and nuanced approach helped ensure that the book reflects the diverse experiences and perspectives of the community. Meghan Howson, my personal assistant, provided the organizational lifeline during the writing process. My American sister-at-heart, Susan Verrilli Dutilh, lent expert input to bring warmth, style, and coherence to the manuscript.

Last, but certainly not least, I am deeply grateful for the unwavering love and support of my family. My parents, Angela and Bruno, who instilled in me the value of hard work and dedication; my husband, Kevin, my biggest cheerleader, sounding board, and constant source of motivation; and our daughter, Lily, whose future I hope will be filled with respect, support, and downright admiration for all women.

Thank you all from the bottom of my heart.

NOTES

CHAPTER 1: YOU ARE NOT CRAZY

Page 5. **1 billion women worldwide:** U.S. Census Bureau, "QuickFacts: United States," https://www.census.gov/quickfacts/fact/table/US/LFE046219.

Page 7. **fewer than one in five ob-gyn residents:** Mindy S. Christianson, Jennifer A. Ducie, Kristiina Altman, et al., "Menopause Education: Needs Assessment of American Obstetrics and Gynecology Residents," *Menopause* 20, no. 11 (2013): 1120–25.

Page 9. **men of the same age do not:** Lisa Mosconi, Valentina Berti, Crystal Quinn, et al., "Sex Differences in Alzheimer Risk: Brain Imaging of Endocrine vs Chronologic Aging," *Neurology* 89, no. 13 (2017): 1382–90.

Page 9. **overall brain chemistry:** Lisa Mosconi, Valentina Berti, Jonathan Dyke, et al., "Menopause Impacts Human Brain Structure, Connectivity, Energy Metabolism, and Amyloid-Beta Deposition," *Scientific Reports* 11 (2021), article 10867.

CHAPTER 2: BUSTING THE BIAS AGAINST WOMEN AND MENOPAUSE

Page 14. **a man attains a higher eminence:** Charles Darwin, *The Descent of Man, and Selection in Relation to Sex* (London: John Murray, 1871).

Page 14. **a marked inferiority of intellectual power:** George J. Romanes, "Mental Differences of Men and Women," *Popular Science Monthly* 31 (1887).

Page 15. **women's brains do differ from men's:** Larry Cahill, "Why Sex Matters for Neuroscience," *Nature Reviews Neuroscience* 7 (2006): 477–84.

Page 16. **women would stop having menstrual discharge:** Grace E. Kohn, Katherine M. Rodriguez, and Alexander W. Pastuszak, "The History of Estrogen Therapy," *Sexual Medicine Reviews* 7, no. 3 (2019): 416–21.

Page 17. **"death of sex":** Susan Mattern, *The Slow Moon Climbs: The Science, History, and Meaning of Menopause* (Princeton, NJ: Princeton University Press, 2019).

Page 17. **were wrongly diagnosed as "crazy":** Rodney J. Baber and J. Wright, "A Brief History of the International Menopause Society," *Climacteric* 20, no. 2 (2017): 85–90.

Page 18. **updating the definition of menopause:** Kohn, Rodriguez, and Pastuszak, "The History of Estrogen Therapy."

Page 18. **calling menopausal women "crippled castrates":** Robert A. Wilson, *Feminine Forever* (New York: M. Evans, 1966).

Page 19. **key not just for reproduction:** Bruce S. McEwen, Stephen E. Alves, Karen Bulloch, and Nancy Weiland," Ovarian Steroids and the Brain: Implications for Cognition and Aging," *Neurology* 48, suppl. 7 (1997): 8S–15S.

Page 19. **deny women of childbearing potential:** E. L. Kinney, J. Trautmann, J. A. Gold, et al., "Underrepresentation of Women in New Drug Trials," *Annals of Internal Medicine* 95, no. 4 (1981): 495–99.

Page 20. **countless drugs have been put on the market:** Ellen Pinnow, Pellavi Sharma, Ameeta Parekh, et al., "Increasing Participation of Women in Early Phase Clinical Trials Approved by the FDA," *Women's Health Issues* 19, no. 2 (2009): 89–93.

Page 20. **variability in sex hormones:** Tracey J. Shors, "A Trip Down Memory Lane About Sex Differences in the Brain," *Philosophical Transactions of the Royal Society B: Biological Sciences* 371, no. 1688 (2016): 20150124.

Page 20. **crucial to supporting brain health:** Aneela Rahman, Hande Jackson, Hollie Hristov, et al., "Sex and Gender Driven Modifiers of Alzheimer's: The Role for Estrogenic Control Across Age, Race, Medical, and Lifestyle Risks," *Frontiers in Aging Neuroscience* 11 (2019): 315.

Page 20. **some statistics most people aren't familiar with:** Lisa Mosconi, *The XX Brain* (New York: Avery, 2020).

Page 23. **resulting in poorer outcomes:** J. Hector Pope, Tom P. Aufderheide, Robin Ruthazer, et al., "Missed Diagnoses of Acute Cardiac Ischemia in the Emergency Department," *New England Journal of Medicine* 342, no. 16 (2000): 1163–70.

Page 23. **to be told their pain is psychosomatic:** Lanlan Zhang, Elizabeth A. Reynolds Losin, Yoni K. Ashar, et al., "Gender Biases in Estimation of Others' Pain," *Journal of Pain* 22, no. 9 (2021): 1048–59.

CHAPTER 3: THE CHANGE NOBODY PREPARED YOU FOR

Page 29. **formalized in medical textbooks:** Soibán D. Harlow, Margery Gass, Janet E. Hall, et al., "Executive Summary of the Stages of Reproductive Aging Workshop + 10: Addressing the Unfinished Agenda of Staging Reproductive Aging," *Journal of Clinical Endocrinology and Metabolism* 97, no. 4 (2012): 1159–68.

Page 30. **ethnicity, genetics, and lifestyle factors:** Patrizia Monteleone, Giulia Mascagni, Andrea Giannini, Andrea Genazzani, et al., "Symptoms of Menopause—Global Prevalence, Physiology and Implications," *Nature Reviews Endocrinology* 14, no. 4 (2018): 199–215.

Page 30. **the average age at menopause:** Monteleone, Mascagni, Giannini, Genazzani, et al., "Symptoms of Menopause—Global Prevalence, Physiology and Implications."

Page 34. **across the globe is forty-nine:** Monteleone, Mascagni, Giannini, Genazzani, et al., "Symptoms of Menopause—Global Prevalence, Physiology and Implications."

Page 37. **your experience of menopause:** Margaret Lock, "Menopause in Cultural Context," *Experimental Gerontology* 29 (1994): 307–317.

Page 38. **the second most common major surgery:** Elizabeth Casiano Evans, Kristen A. Matteson, Francisco J. Orejuela, et al., "Salpingo-Oophorectomy at the Time of Benign Hysterectomy: A Systematic Review," *Obstetrics and Gynecology* 128, no. 3 (2016): 476–85.

Page 39. **bilateral salpingo-oophorectomy (BSO) is of established clinical benefit:** Evans, Matteson, Orejuela, et al., "Salpingo-Oophorectomy at the Time of Benign Hysterectomy: A Systematic Review."

Page 39. **roughly 90 percent of all hysterectomies:** ACOG Committee Opinion no. 701, "Choosing the Route of Hysterectomy for Benign Disease," *Obstetrics and Gynecology* 129, no. 6 (2017): e155–e159.

Page 39. **common practice to conserve the ovaries:** ACOG Committee Opinion no. 701, "Choosing the Route of Hysterectomy for Benign Disease."

Page 40. **might still lower the risk of heart disease:** William H. Parker, Michael S. Broder, Eunice Chang, et al., "Ovarian Conservation at the Time of Hysterectomy and Long-Term Health Outcomes in the Nurses' Health Study," *Obstetrics & Gynecology* 113, no. 5 (2009): 1027–37.

Page 40. **current guidelines recommend ovarian conservation:** ACOG Committee Opinion no. 701, "Choosing the Route of Hysterectomy for Benign Disease."

Page 40. **over half of all American women undergoing hysterectomies:** Parker, Broder, Chang, et al., "Ovarian Conservation at the Time of Hysterectomy and Long-Term Health Outcomes in the Nurses' Health Study."

Page 40. **Twenty-three percent of American women aged forty to forty-four:** Stephanie S. Faubion, Julia A. Files, and Walter A. Rocca, "Elective Oophorectomy: Primum Non Nocere," *Journal of Women's Health* (Larchmont) 25, no. 2 (2016): 200–202.

CHAPTER 4: MENOPAUSE BRAIN IS NOT JUST YOUR IMAGINATION

Page 43. **10 to 15 percent of women report no changes:** Patrizia Monteleone, Giulia Mascagni, Andrea Giannini, et al., "Symptoms of Menopause—Global Prevalence, Physiology and Implications," *Nature Reviews Endocrinology* 14, no. 4 (2018): 199–215.

Page 45. **Hot flashes are considered:** Monteleone, Mascagni, Giannini, Genazzani, et al., "Symptoms of Menopause—Global Prevalence, Physiology and Implications."

Page 45. **hot flashes for three to five years:** Monteleone, Mascagni, Giannini, Genazzani, et al., "Symptoms of Menopause—Global Prevalence, Physiology and Implications."

Page 45. **four patterns when it comes to hot flashes:** Ping G. Tepper, Maria M. Brooks, John F. Randolph Jr., et al., "Characterizing the Trajectories of Vasomotor Symptoms Across the Menopausal Transition," *Menopause* 23, no. 10 (2016): 1067–74.

Page 46. **they tend to occur frequently:** Monteleone, Mascagni, Giannini, Genazzani, et al., "Symptoms of Menopause—Global Prevalence, Physiology and Implications."

Page 47. **women who experience hot flashes earlier in life:** Rebecca C. Thurston, Yuefang Chang, Emma Barinas-Mitchell, et al., "Physiologically Assessed Hot Flashes and Endothelial Function Among Midlife Women," *Menopause* 25, no. 11 (2018): 1354–61.

Page 47. **linked to white-matter lesions in the brain:** Rebecca C. Thurston, Howard J. Aizenstein, Carol A. Derby, et al., "Menopausal Hot Flashes and White Matter Hyperintensities," *Menopause* 23, no. 1 (2016): 27–32.

Page 47. **Roughly 20 percent of all women experience mood swings:** Katherine M. Reding, Peter J. Schmidt, and David R. Rubinow, "Perimenopausal Depression and Early Menopause: Cause or Consequence?" *Menopause* 24, no. 12 (2017): 1333–35.

Page 49. **sleep is essential in forming memories:** Adam J. Krause, Eti Ben Simon, Bryce A. Mander, et al., "The Sleep-Deprived Human Brain," *Nature Reviews Neuroscience* 18, no. 7 (2017): 404–18.

Page 49. **report more sleep issues:** NIH State-of-the-Science Panel, "National Institutes of Health State-of-the-Science Conference Statement: Management of Menopause-Related Symptoms," *Annals of Internal Medicine* 142 (2005): 1003–13.

Page 49. **more likely than other people to report spin-off problems:** Eric Suni and Nilong Vyas, "How Is Sleep Different for Men and Women?" National Sleep Foundation, updated March 7, 2023, https://www.sleepfoundation.org /how-sleep-works/how-is-sleep-different-for-men-and-women.

Page 49. **According to the Centers for Disease Control and Prevention:** Anjel Vahratian, "Sleep Duration and Quality Among Women Aged 40–59, by Menopausal Status," National Center for Health Statistics Data Brief No. 286, September 2017, https://www.cdc.gov/nchs/products/databriefs /db286.htm.

Page 49. **Sleep apnea is a chronic breathing disorder:** Martin R. Cowie, "Sleep Apnea: State of the Art," *Trends in Cardiovascular Medicine* 27, no. 4 (2017): 280–89.

Page 49. **a partial or complete obstruction:** Cowie, "Sleep Apnea: State of the Art."

Page 51. **over 60 percent of all perimenopausal and postmenopausal women:** Gail A. Greendale, Arun S. Karlamangla, and Pauline M. Maki, "The Menopause Transition and Cognition," *JAMA* 323, no. 15 (2020): 1495–96.

Page 51. **forgetfulness can spike:** Ellen B. Gold, Barbara Sternfeld, Jennifer L. Kelsey, et al., "Relation of Demographic and Lifestyle Factors to Symptoms in a Multi-Racial/Ethnic Population of Women 40–55 Years of Age," *American Journal of Epidemiology* 152, no. 5 (2000): 463–73.

Page 52. **objectively within the appropriate reference range:** Pauline M. Maki and Victor W. Henderson, "Cognition and the Menopause Transition," *Menopause* 23, no. 7 (2016): 803–805.

Page 53. **scores on some cognitive tests:** Gail A. Greendale, M-H. Huang, R. G. Wight, et al., "Effects of the Menopause Transition and Hormone Use on Cognitive Performance in Midlife Women," *Neurology* 72, no. 21 (2009): 1850–57.

Page 54. **true both *before and after* menopause:** Dorene M. Rentz, Blair K. Weiss, Emily G. Jacobs, et al., "Sex Differences in Episodic Memory in Early Midlife: Impact of Reproductive Aging," *Menopause* 24, no. 4 (2017): 400–408.

Page 55. **women are two to three times more likely:** Jan L. Shifren, Brigitta U. Monz, Patricia A. Russo, et al., "Sexual Problems and Distress in United States Women: Prevalence and Correlates," *Obstetrics & Gynecology* 112, no. 5 (2008): 970–78.

Page 55. **as many as 20 percent of women:** Shifren, Monz, Russo, et al., "Sexual Problems and Distress in United States Women: Prevalence and Correlates."

Page 55. **during the late postmenopausal phase:** Shifren, Monz, Russo, et al., "Sexual Problems and Distress in United States Women: Prevalence and Correlates."

Page 56. **rate how important sex was to them:** Nancy E. Avis, Sarah Brockwell, John F. Randolph, et al., "Longitudinal Changes in Sexual Functioning as Women Transition Through Menopause: Results from the Study of Women's Health Across the Nation," *Menopause* 16, no. 3 (2009): 442–52.

CHAPTER 5: BRAIN AND OVARIES: PARTNERS IN TIME

Page 62. **intricately wired for reproduction:** Lisa Yang, Alexander N. Comninos, and Waljit S. Dhillo, "Intrinsic Links Among Sex, Emotion, and Reproduction," *Cellular and Molecular Life Sciences* 75, no. 12 (2018): 2197–210.

Page 65. **estrogen in particular has been shown to boost a woman's metabolism:** Eugenia Morselli, Roberta de Souza Santos, Alfredo Criollo, et al., "The Effects of Oestrogens and Their Receptors on Cardiometabolic Health," *Nature Reviews Endocrinology* 13, no. 6 (2017): 352–64.

Page 65. **instrumental in maintaining bone health:** Stavros C. Manolagas, Charles A. O'Brien, and Maria Almeida, "The Role of Estrogen and Androgen Receptors in Bone Health and Disease," *Nature Reviews Endocrinology* 9, no. 12 (2013): 699–712.

Page 65. **keeping tabs on inflammation and cholesterol levels:** Morselli, Santos, Criollo, et al., "The Effects of Oestrogens and Their Receptors on Cardiometabolic Health."

Page 69. **the title of master regulator of the female brain:** Jamaica A. Rettberg, Jia Yao, and Roberta Diaz Brinton, "Estrogen: A Master Regulator of Bioenergetic Systems in the Brain and Body," *Frontiers in Neuroendocrinology* 35, no. 1 (2014): 8–30.

Page 69. **Neuroprotection:** Deena Khan and S. Ansar Ahmed, "The Immune System Is a Natural Target for Estrogen Action: Opposing Effects of Estrogen in Two Prototypical Autoimmune Diseases," *Frontiers in Immunology* 6 (2015): 635.

Page 70. *neurotransmitters*, **the brain's chemical messengers:** Claudia Barth, Arno Villringer, and Julia Sacher," Sex Hormones Affect Neurotransmitters and Shape the Adult Female Brain During Hormonal Transition Periods," *Frontiers in Neuroscience* 9 (2015): 37.

Page 70. **Protection. Estradiol supports the immune system:** Sandra Zárate, Tinna Stevnsner, and Ricardo Gredilla, "Role of Estrogen and Other Sex Hormones in Brain Aging. Neuroprotection and DNA Repair," *Frontiers in Aging Neuroscience* 9 (2017): 430.

Page 73. **the energy changes appeared to be** *temporary:* Lisa Mosconi, Valentina Berti, Jonathan Dyke, et al., "Menopause Impacts Human Brain Structure, Connectivity, Energy Metabolism, and Amyloid-Beta Deposition," *Scientific Reports* 11 (2021): article 10867.

Page 73. **appeared to plateau for quite a few women:** Mosconi, Berti, Dyke, et al., "Menopause Impacts Human Brain Structure, Connectivity, Energy Metabolism, and Amyloid-Beta Deposition."

CHAPTER 6: PUTTING MENOPAUSE IN CONTEXT: THE THREE P'S

Page 76. **all children's brains appear exactly the same:** T. Beking, R. H. Geuze, M. van Faassen, et al., "Prenatal and Pubertal Testosterone Affect Brain Lateralization," *Psychoneuroendocrinology* 88 (2018): 78–91.

Page 77. **estrogen and testosterone play an essential role in the sexual differentiation of the brain:** Larry Cahill, "Why Sex Matters for Neuroscience," *Nature Reviews Neuroscience* 7, no. 6 (2006): 477–84.

Page 77. **80 to 100 billion nerve cells:** Robin Gibb and Bryan Kolb, eds., *The Neurobiology of Brain and Behavioral Development,* 1st ed. (Boston: Elsevier, 2017).

Page 78. **about half of the brain's original neurons:** Sarah-Jayne Blakemore, "The Social Brain in Adolescence," *Nature Reviews Neuroscience* 9, no. 4 (2008): 267–77.

Page 78. **changes developing at varying rates:** Jay N. Giedd, Jonathan Blumenthal, Neal O. Jeffries, et al., "Brain Development During Childhood and Adolescence: A Longitudinal MRI Study," *Nature Neuroscience* 2, no. 10 (1999): 861–63.

Page 78. **a frontal cortex still under construction:** Sarah-Jayne Blakemore and Trevor W. Robbins, "Decision-Making in the Adolescent Brain," *Nature Neuroscience* 15 (2012): 1184–91.

Page 79. **the puberty-fueled brain revamp:** Blakemore, "The Social Brain in Adolescence."

Page 79. **the brain maturation timeline:** Giedd, Blumenthal, Jeffries, et al., "Brain Development During Childhood and Adolescence: A Longitudinal MRI Study."

Page 79. **girls tend to exhibit earlier and stronger connections:** Nitin Gogtay, Jay N. Giedd, Leslie Lusk, et al., "Dynamic Mapping of Human Cortical Development During Childhood Through Early Adulthood," *PNAS* 101, no. 21 (2004): 8174–79.

Page 79. **evidence that girls mature faster than boys:** Cecilia I. Calero, Alejo Salles, Mariano Semelman, and Mariano Sigman, "Age and Gender Dependent Development of Theory of Mind in 6- to 8-Years Old Children," *Frontiers in Human Neuroscience* 7 (2013): 281.

Page 79. **empathy:** Simon Baron-Cohen, Rebecca C. Knickmeyer, and Matthew K. Belmonte, "Sex Differences in the Brain: Implications for Explaining Autism," *Science* 310, no. 5749 (2005): 819–23.

Page 79. **social competence skills, and social understanding:** Sandra Bosacki, Flavia Pissoto Moreira, Valentina Sitnik, et al., "Theory of Mind, Self-Knowledge, and Perceptions of Loneliness in Emerging Adolescents," *Journal of Genetic Psychology* 181, no. 1 (2020): 14–31.

Page 79. **better communication abilities:** Baron-Cohen, Knickmeyer, and Belmonte, "Sex Differences in the Brain: Implications for Explaining Autism."

Page 80. **brain cells visibly sprout:** C. S. Woolley and B. S. McEwen, "Estradiol Mediates Fluctuation in Hippocampal Synapse Density During the Estrous Cycle in the Adult Rat," *Journal of Neuroscience* 12, no. 7 (1992): 2549–54.

Page 80. **amygdala and hippocampus swell appreciably in size:** Claudia Barth, Christopher J. Steele, Karsten Mueller, et al., "In-Vivo Dynamics of the Human Hippocampus Across the Menstrual Cycle," *Scientific Reports* 6, no. 1 (2016): 32833.

Page 80. **connections with the prefrontal cortex appear to get stronger:** Manon Dubol, C. Neill Epperson, Julia Sacher, et al., "Neuroimaging the Menstrual Cycle: A Multimodal Systematic Review," *Frontiers in Neuroendocrinology* 60 (2021): 100878.

Page 80. **Certain cognitive skills are also heightened:** Pauline M. Maki, Jill B. Rich, and R. Shayna Rosenbaum, "Implicit Memory Varies Across the Menstrual

Cycle: Estrogen Effects in Young Women," *Neuropsychologia* 40, no. 5 (2002): 518–29.

Page 80. **linked to low mood, irritability:** Kimberly Ann Yonkers, P. M. Shaughn O'Brien, and Elias Eriksson, "Premenstrual Syndrome," *Lancet* 371, no. 9619 (2008): 1200–10.

Page 80. **shifts from being equal between girls and boys before puberty:** Tomáš Paus, Matcheri Keshavan, and Jay N. Giedd, "Why Do Many Psychiatric Disorders Emerge During Adolescence?" *Nature Reviews Neuroscience* 9 (2008): 947–57.

Page 80. **one out of four women suffers from clinical PMS:** L. J. Baker and P. M. S. O'Brien, "Premenstrual Syndrome (PMS): A Peri-Menopausal Perspective," *Maturitas* 72, no. 2 (2012): 121–25.

Page 81. **they can be severe:** Yonkers, O'Brien, and Eriksson, "Premenstrual Syndrome."

Page 81. **come into adulthood gifted:** David I. Miller and Diane F. Halpern, "The New Science of Cognitive Sex Differences," *Trends in Cognitive Science* 18, no. 1 (2014): 37–45.

Page 81. **as well as episodic memory:** Martin Asperholm, Sanket Nagar, Serhiy Dekhtyar, and Agneta Herlitz, "The Magnitude of Sex Differences in Verbal Episodic Memory Increases with Social Progress: Data from 54 Countries Across 40 Years," *PLoS One* 14, no. 4 (2019): e0214945.

Page 81. **rise and fall with each of our menstrual cycles:** Sara N. Burke and Carol A. Barnes, "Neural Plasticity in the Ageing Brain," *Nature Reviews Neuroscience* 7 (2006): 30–40.

Page 82. **researchers did brain scans on twenty-five first-time mothers:** Elseline Hoekzema, Erika Barba-Müller, Cristina Pozzobon, et al., "Pregnancy Leads to Long-Lasting Changes in Human Brain Structure," *Nature Neuroscience* 20, no. 2 (2017): 287–96.

Page 83. **pregnancy triggers a comparable development:** Hoekzema, Barba-Müller, Pozzobon, et al., "Pregnancy Leads to Long-Lasting Changes in Human Brain Structure."

Page 84. **The hippocampus and the amygdala had actually *grown back*:** Hoekzema, Barba-Müller, Pozzobon, et al., "Pregnancy Leads to Long-Lasting Changes in Human Brain Structure."

Page 84. **The frontal cortex also displayed:** Eileen Luders, Florian Kurth, Malin Gingnell, et al., "From Baby Brain to Mommy Brain: Widespread Gray Matter Gain After Giving Birth," *Cortex* 126 (2020): 334–42.

Page 84. **mothers can recognize their little ones *by scent*:** M. Kaitz, A. Good, A. M. Rokem, and A. I. Eidelman, "Mothers' Recognition of Their Newborns by Olfactory Cues," *Developmental Psychobiology* 20, no. 6 (1987): 587–91.

Page 84. **release copious amounts of *oxytocin*:** Megan Galbally, Andrew James Lewis, Marinus van Ijzendoorn, and Michael Permezel, "The Role of Oxytocin in Mother-Infant Relations: A Systematic Review of Human Studies," *Harvard Review of Psychiatry* 19, no. 1 (2011): 1–14.

Page 85. ***maternal aggression*:** Oliver J. Bosch, Simone L. Meddle, Daniela I. Beiderbeck, et al., "Brain Oxytocin Correlates with Maternal Aggression: Link to Anxiety," *Journal of Neuroscience* 25, no. 29 (2005): 6807–15.

Page 86. **over 80 percent of pregnant women perceive a decline:** Peter M. Brindle, Malcolm W. Brown, John Brown, et al., "Objective and Subjective Memory Impairment in Pregnancy," *Psychological Medicine* 21, no. 3 (1991): 647–53.

Page 86. **almost half of all new mothers experiencing forgetfulness:** Ashleigh J. Filtness, Janelle MacKenzie, and Kerry Armstrong, "Longitudinal Change in

Sleep and Daytime Sleepiness in Postpartum Women," *PLoS One* 9, no. 7 (2014): e103513.

Page 86. **can indeed be impacted by pregnancy and postpartum:** Sasha J. Davies, Jarrad AG Lum, Helen Skouteris, et al., "Cognitive Impairment During Pregnancy: A Meta-Analysis," *Medical Journal of Australia* 208, no. 1 (2018): 35–40.

Page 87. **these changes are temporary:** Hoekzema, Barba-Müller, Pozzobon, et al., "Pregnancy Leads to Long-Lasting Changes in Human Brain Structure."

Page 87. **their IQ is unquestionably unaltered:** Helen Christensen, Liana S. Leach, and Andrew Mackinnon, "Cognition in Pregnancy and Motherhood: Prospective Cohort Study," *British Journal of Psychiatry* 196, no. 2 (2010): 126–32.

Page 88. **more likely to experience altered mood:** Ellen W. Freeman, "Treatment of Depression Associated with the Menstrual Cycle: Premenstrual Dysphoria, Postpartum Depression, and the Perimenopause," *Dialogues in Clinical Neuroscience* 4, no. 2 (2002): 177–91.

Page 88. **About one in every eight new moms:** Katherine L. Wisner, Barbara L. Parry, and Catherine M. Piontek, "Clinical Practice. Postpartum Depression," *New England Journal of Medicine* 347, no. 3 (2002): 194–99.

Page 88. **mothers suffering from postpartum depression:** Ian Brockington, "A Historical Perspective on the Psychiatry of Motherhood," in A. Riecher-Rössler and M. Steiner, eds., *Perinatal Stress, Mood and Anxiety Disorders: From Bench to Bedside*, Bibliotheca Psychiatrica No. 173 (Basel, Switzerland: Karger Publishers, 2005), 1–6.

CHAPTER 7: THE UPSIDE OF MENOPAUSE

Page 93. **hot flashes are another symptom:** Rebecca C. Thurston, James F. Luther, Stephen R. Wisniewski, et al., "Prospective Evaluation of Nighttime Hot Flashes During Pregnancy and Postpartum," *Fertility and Sterility* 100, no. 6 (2013): 1667–72.

Page 96. **postmenopausal women report improved mood:** Katherine E. Campbell, Lorraine Dennerstein, Mark Tacey, and Cassandra E. Szoeke, "The Trajectory of Negative Mood and Depressive Symptoms over Two Decades," *Maturitas* 95 (2017): 36–41.

Page 96. **62 percent stating that they felt:** Lotte Hvas, "Positive Aspects of Menopause: A Qualitative Study," *Maturitas* 39, no. 1 (2001): 11–17.

Page 96. **65 percent of British postmenopausal women:** Social Issues Research Centre, "Jubilee Women. Fiftysomething Women—Lifestyle and Attitudes Now and Fifty Years Ago," http://www.sirc.org/publik/jubilee _women.pdf.

Page 97. **climbs to new heights later in life:** Arthur A. Stone, Joseph E. Schwartz, Joan E. Broderick, and Angus Deaton, "A Snapshot of the Age Distribution of Psychological Well-Being in the United States," *PNAS* 107, no. 22 (2010): 9985–90.

Page 97. **Increase in mood and optimism:** Campbell, Dennerstein, Tacey, and Szoeke, "The Trajectory of Negative Mood and Depressive Symptoms over Two Decades."

Page 98. **frequently cited as one of the utmost benefits of menopause:** Nancy E. Avis, Alicia Colvin, Arun S. Karlamangla, et al., "Change in Sexual Functioning over the Menopausal Transition: Results from the Study of

Women's Health Across the Nation (SWAN)," *Menopause* 24, no. 4 (2017): 379–90.

Page 98. **only too happy to have more me time:** Campbell, Dennerstein, Tacey, and Szoeke, "The Trajectory of Negative Mood and Depressive Symptoms over Two Decades."

Page 99. **the capacity to sustain joy, wonder, and gratitude often increases:** Lotte Hvas, "Menopausal Women's Positive Experience of Growing Older," *Maturitas* 54, no. 3 (2006): 245–51.

Page 100. **the postmenopausal amygdala is less responsive:** Mara Mather, Turhan Canli, Tammy English, et al., "Amygdala Responses to Emotionally Valenced Stimuli in Older and Younger Adults," *Psychological Science* 15, no. 4 (2004): 259–63.

Page 100. **activate their rational prefrontal cortex more:** Alison Berent-Spillson, Courtney Marsh, Carol Persad, et al., "Metabolic and Hormone Influences on Emotion Processing During Menopause," *Psychoneuroendocrinology* 76 (2017): 218–25.

Page 100. **women in their fifties show greater empathy:** Ed O'Brien, Sara H. Konrath, Daniel Grühn, and Anna Linda Hagen, "Empathic Concern and Perspective Taking: Linear and Quadratic Effects of Age Across the Adult Life Span," *Journals of Gerontology, Series B, Psychological Sciences and Social Sciences* 68, no. 2 (2013): 168–75.

Page 100. **empathic concern or sympathy continues to increase:** Cornelia Wieck and Ute Kunzmann, "Age Differences in Empathy: Multidirectional and Context-Dependent," *Psychology and Aging* 30, no. 2 (2015): 407–19.

Page 101. **grandmothers' emotional reactions:** James K. Rilling, Amber Gonzalez, and Minwoo Lee, "The Neural Correlates of Grandmaternal Caregiving," *Proceedings of the Royal Society B: Biological Sciences* 288, no. 1963 (2021): 20211997.

CHAPTER 8: THE WHY OF MENOPAUSE

Page 104. **the evolutionary mismatch hypothesis:** Alan A. Cohen, "Female Post-Reproductive Lifespan: A General Mammalian Trait," *Biological Reviews of the Cambridge Philosophical Society* 79, no. 4 (2004): 733–50.

Page 105. **grandma is doing much of the work:** Hillard Kaplan, Michael Gurven, Jeffrey Winking, et al., "Learning, Menopause, and the Human Adaptive Complex," *Annals of the New York Academy of Sciences* 1204 (2010): 30–42.

Page 105. **grandmother hypothesis:** Kristen Hawkes, "Human Longevity: The Grandmother Effect," *Nature* 428, no. 6979 (2004): 128–29.

Page 106. **carrying grandma's longevity genes:** Mike Takahashi, Rama S. Singh, and John Stone, "A Theory for the Origin of Human Menopause," *Frontiers in Genetics* 7 (2016): 222.

Page 106. **every female *Homo sapiens* carried DNA:** Kristen Hawkes, James F. O'Connell, Nicholas Blurton-Jones, et al., "Grandmothering, Menopause, and the Evolution of Human Life Histories," *PNAS* 95, no. 3 (1998): 1336–39.

Page 106. **research on killer whales:** Michael A. Cant and Rufus A. Johnstone, "Reproductive Conflict and the Separation of Reproductive Generations in Humans," *PNAS* 105, no. 14 (2008): 5332–36.

Page 107. **As humans, we distinguish ourselves:** Sarah Blaffer Hrdy and Judith M. Burkart, "The Emergence of Emotionally Modern Humans: Implications for Language and Learning," *Philosophical Transactions of the Royal Society B: Biological Sciences* 375 (2020): 20190499.

CHAPTER 9: ESTROGEN THERAPY FOR MENOPAUSE

Page 113. **women on HRT reported having fewer hot flashes:** F. Grodstein, J. E. Manson, G. A. Colditz, et al., "A Prospective, Observational Study of Postmenopausal Hormone Therapy and Primary Prevention of Cardiovascular Disease," *Annals of Internal Medicine* 133, no. 12 (2000): 933–41.

Page 114. **women on hormones had *more* heart trouble:** Jacques E. Rossouw, Garnet L. Anderson, Ross L. Prentice, et al., "Risks and Benefits of Estrogen Plus Progestin in Healthy Postmenopausal Women: Principal Results from the Women's Health Initiative Randomized Controlled Trial," *JAMA* 288, no. 3 (2002): 321–33.

Page 114. **risk for blood clots and breast cancer:** Garnet L. Anderson, Howard L. Judd, Andrew M. Kaunitz, et al., "Effects of Estrogen Plus Progestin on Gynecologic Cancers and Associated Diagnostic Procedures: The Women's Health Initiative Randomized Trial," *JAMA* 290, no. 13 (2003): 1739–48.

Page 114. **risk of dementia had gone up:** Sally A. Shumaker, Claudine Legault, Stephen R. Rapp, et al., "Estrogen Plus Progestin and the Incidence of Dementia and Mild Cognitive Impairment in Postmenopausal Women: The Women's Health Initiative Memory Study: A Randomized Controlled Trial," *JAMA* 289, no. 20 (2003): 2651–62.

Page 115. **risk of breast cancer was increased only for the women taking the estrogen-plus-progestin:** Garnet L. Anderson, Marian Limacher, Annlouise R. Assaf, et al., "Effects of Conjugated Equine Estrogen in Postmenopausal Women with Hysterectomy: The Women's Health Initiative Randomized Controlled Trial," *JAMA* 291, no. 14 (2004): 1701–12.

Page 115. **23 percent *reduced* occurrence of breast cancer:** Andrea Z. LaCroix, Rowan T. Chlebowski, JoAnn E. Manson, et al., "Health Outcomes After Stopping Conjugated Equine Estrogens Among Postmenopausal Women with Prior Hysterectomy: A Randomized Controlled Trial," *JAMA* 305 (2011): 1305–14.

Page 116. **oral estradiol may be safer than oral CEEs:** Chrisandra L. Shufelt and JoAnn E. Manson, "Menopausal Hormone Therapy and Cardiovascular Disease: The Role of Formulation, Dose, and Route of Delivery," *Journal of Clinical Endocrinology and Metabolism* 106, no. 5 (2021): 1245–1254.

Page 116. **observational data suggest that it is less risky:** Shufelt and Manson, "Menopausal Hormone Therapy and Cardiovascular Disease: The Role of Formulation, Dose, and Route of Delivery."

Page 117. **a factor in promoting breast cancer:** Rossouw, Anderson, Prentice, et al., "Risks and Benefits of Estrogen Plus Progestin in Healthy Postmenopausal Women: Principal Results from the Women's Health Initiative Randomized Controlled Trial."

Page 117. **bioidentical progesterone does not increase the risk of breast cancer:** Shufelt and Manson, "Menopausal Hormone Therapy and Cardiovascular Disease: The Role of Formulation, Dose, and Route of Delivery."

Page 118. **HRT works best while our bodies:** Roberta Diaz Brinton, "The Healthy Cell Bias of Estrogen Action: Mitochondrial Bioenergetics and Neurological Implications," *Trends in Neurosciences* 31, no. 10 (2008): 529–37.

Page 120. **HRT started at the right time:** John H. Morrison, Roberta D. Brinton, Peter J. Schmidt, and Andrea C. Gore, "Estrogen, Menopause, and the Aging Brain: How Basic Neuroscience Can Inform Hormone Therapy in Women," *Journal of Neuroscience* 26, no. 41 (2006): 10332–48.

Page 121. **HRT was associated with a *reduced* risk of heart attacks:** Shelley R. Salpeter, Ji Cheng, Lehana Thabane, et al., "Bayesian Meta-Analysis of Hormone Therapy and Mortality in Younger Postmenopausal Women," *American Journal of Medicine* 122, no. 11 (2009): 1016–1022.e1011.

Page 121. **an overall lower mortality rate than those who did not take hormones:** JoAnn E. Manson, Aaron K. Aragaki, Jacques E. Rossouw, et al., "Menopausal Hormone Therapy and Long-Term All-Cause and Cause-Specific Mortality: The Women's Health Initiative Randomized Trials," *JAMA* 318 (2017): 927–38.

Page 121. **the North American Menopause Society:** NAMS 2022 Hormone Therapy Position Statement Advisory Panel, "The 2022 Hormone Therapy Position Statement of the North American Menopause Society," *Menopause* 29, no. 7 (2022): 767–94.

Page 122. **the mortality rate of women taking hormones was no higher:** Anderson, Limacher, Assaf, et al., "Effects of Conjugated Equine Estrogen in Postmenopausal Women with Hysterectomy: The Women's Health Initiative Randomized Controlled Trial."

Page 122. **hysterectomies resulted in 7 *fewer* breast cancer cases:** LaCroix, Chlebowski, Manson, et al., "Health Outcomes After Stopping Conjugated Equine Estrogens Among Postmenopausal Women with Prior Hysterectomy: A Randomized Controlled Trial."

Page 122. **current guidelines defining it as a "rare occurrence":** NAMS 2022 Hormone Therapy Position Statement Advisory Panel, "The 2022 Hormone Therapy Position Statement of the North American Menopause Society."

Page 122. **risk of cancer reoccurrence remains a concern:** Collaborative Group on Hormonal Factors in Breast Cancer, "Type and Timing of Menopausal Hormone Therapy and Breast Cancer Risk: Individual Participant Meta-Analysis of the Worldwide Epidemiological Evidence," *Lancet* 394, no. 10204 (2019): 1159–68.

Page 123. **carries a similar risk of breast cancer as:** Roger A. Lobo, "Hormone-Replacement Therapy: Current Thinking," *Nature Reviews Endocrinology* 13, no. 4 (2017): 220–31.

Page 123. **two glasses of wine per day or being significantly overweight increases the risk:** Lobo, "Hormone-Replacement Therapy: Current Thinking."

Page 123. **that position may have been inadequate:** NAMS 2022 Hormone Therapy Position Statement Advisory Panel, "The 2022 Hormone Therapy Position Statement of the North American Menopause Society."

Page 124. **the data no longer support that cutoff:** "Joint Position Statement by the British Menopause Society, Royal College of Obstetricians and Gynaecologists and Society for Endocrinology on Best Practice Recommendations for the Care of Women Experiencing the Menopause," https://www.endocrinology.org/media/d3pbn14o/joint-position-statement-on-best-practice-recommendations-for-the-care-of-women-experiencing-the-menopause.pdf.

Page 124. **hormone therapy is actually recommended:** NAMS 2022 Hormone Therapy Position Statement Advisory Panel, "The 2022 Hormone Therapy Position Statement of the North American Menopause Society."

Page 124. **patients should be encouraged to start HRT:** NAMS 2022 Hormone Therapy Position Statement Advisory Panel, "The 2022 Hormone Therapy Position Statement of the North American Menopause Society."

Page 125. **If HRT is to be started after age sixty:** NAMS 2022 Hormone Therapy Position Statement Advisory Panel, "The 2022 Hormone Therapy Position Statement of the North American Menopause Society."

Page 125. **vaginal estrogen can be started at any age:** NAMS 2022 Hormone Therapy Position Statement Advisory Panel, "The 2022 Hormone Therapy Position Statement of the North American Menopause Society."

Page 126. **estrogen-alone and estrogen-plus-progestin regimens reduced the number of hot flashes:** NAMS 2022 Hormone Therapy Position Statement Advisory Panel, "The 2022 Hormone Therapy Position Statement of the North American Menopause Society."

Page 127. **low-dose estrogen with or without progesterone may reduce sleep disturbances:** NAMS 2022 Hormone Therapy Position Statement Advisory Panel, "The 2022 Hormone Therapy Position Statement of the North American Menopause Society."

Page 127. **mild depressive symptoms associated with perimenopause:** David R. Rubinow, Sarah Lanier Johnson, Peter J. Schmidt, et al., "Efficacy of Estradiol in Perimenopausal Depression: So Much Promise and So Few Answers," *Depression & Anxiety Journal* 32, no. 8 (2015): 539–49.

Page 128. **can support and even enhance some aspects of cognition:** Pauline M. Maki and Erin Sundermann, "Hormone Therapy and Cognitive Function," *Human Reproduction Update* 15, no. 6 (2009): 667–81.

Page 128. **particularly evident for those undergoing hysterectomy:** Steven Jett, Eva Schelbaum, Grace Jang, et al., "Ovarian Steroid Hormones: A Long Overlooked but Critical Contributor to Brain Aging and Alzheimer's Disease," *Frontiers in Aging Neuroscience* 14 (2022): 948219.

Page 128. **no effects or even detrimental effects depending on the type of HRT:** Jett, Schelbaum, Jang, et al., "Ovarian Steroid Hormones: A Long Overlooked but Critical Contributor to Brain Aging and Alzheimer's Disease."

Page 129. **those taking estrogen in midlife didn't develop dementia:** Erin S. LeBlanc, Jeri Janowsky, Benjamin K. S. Chan, and Heidi D. Nelson, "Hormone Replacement Therapy and Cognition: Systematic Review and Meta-Analysis," *JAMA* 285 (2001): 1489–99.

Page 129. **Several observational studies report similar findings:** Brinton, "The Healthy Cell Bias of Estrogen Action: Mitochondrial Bioenergetics and Neurological Implications."

Page 130. **does not increase the risk of breast or uterine cancer:** Lon S. Schneider, Gerson Hernandez, Ligin Zhao, et al., "Safety and Feasibility of Estrogen Receptor-Beta Targeted PhytoSERM Formulation for Menopausal Symptoms: Phase 1b/2a Randomized Clinical Trial," *Menopause* 26 (2019): 874–84.

CHAPTER 10: OTHER HORMONAL AND NONHORMONAL THERAPIES

Page 134. **with aging, testosterone does decline:** Rebecca Glaser and Constantine Dimitrakakis, "Testosterone Therapy in Women: Myths and Misconceptions," *Maturitas* 74, no. 3 (2013): 230–34.

Page 134. **Women with low testosterone levels:** Glaser and Dimitrakakis, "Testosterone Therapy in Women: Myths and Misconceptions."

Page 135. **testosterone therapy can be effective to increase sexual desire:** Rakibul M. Islam, Robin J. Bell, Sally Green, et al., "Safety and Efficacy of Testosterone for Women: A Systematic Review and Meta-Analysis of

Randomised Controlled Trial Data," *Lancet Diabetes & Endocrinology* 7, no. 10 (2019): 754–66.

Page 135. **According to current guidelines:** NAMS 2022 Hormone Therapy Position Statement Advisory Panel, "The 2022 Hormone Therapy Position Statement of the North American Menopause Society," *Menopause* 29, no. 7 (2022): 767–94.

Page 135. **to improve mood or cognition:** NAMS 2022 Hormone Therapy Position Statement Advisory Panel, "The 2022 Hormone Therapy Position Statement of the North American Menopause Society."

Page 135. **the available evidence is very limited:** Susan R. Davis, Sonia L. Davison, Maria Gavrilescu, et al., "Effects of Testosterone on Visuospatial Function and Verbal Fluency in Postmenopausal Women: Results from a Functional Magnetic Resonance Imaging Pilot Study," *Menopause* 21 (2014): 410–14.

Page 136. **improvement in some aspects of cognition:** Susan R. Davis and Sarah Wahlin-Jacobsen, "Testosterone in Women—The Clinical Significance," *Lancet Diabetes & Endocrinology* 3, no. 12 (2015): 980–92.

Page 136. **just as many small studies have reported no improvement:** Davis and Wahlin-Jacobsen, "Testosterone in Women—The Clinical Significance."

Page 136. **hair loss, acne, and hirsutism:** Davis and Wahlin-Jacobsen, "Testosterone in Women—The Clinical Significance."

Page 137. **low-dose oral contraceptives can reduce:** A. M. Kaunitz, "Oral Contraceptive Use in Perimenopause," *American Journal of Obstetrics & Gynecology* 185, suppl. 2 (2001): S32–37.

Page 137. **reduction in vasomotor symptoms:** July Guerin, Alexandra Engelmann, Meena Mattamana, and Laura M. Borgelt, "Use of Hormonal Contraceptives in Perimenopause: A Systematic Review," *Pharmacotherapy* 42 (2022): 154–64.

Page 137. **a reduced risk of developing endometrial and ovarian cancer:** Kaunitz, "Oral Contraceptive Use in Perimenopause."

Page 138. **a higher chance of starting antidepressants:** Charlotte Wessel Skovlund, Lina Steinrud Mørch, Lars Vedel Kessing, and Øjvind Lidegaard, "Association of Hormonal Contraception with Depression," *JAMA Psychiatry* 73, no. 11 (2016): 1154–62.

Page 138. **hormonal contraception may be helpful as an alternative form:** Jett, Malviya, Schelbaum, et al., "Endogenous and Exogenous Estrogen Exposures: How Women's Reproductive Health Can Drive Brain Aging and Inform Alzheimer's Prevention."

Page 140. **reduce hot flashes by 20 to 60 percent:** "Nonhormonal Management of Menopause-Associated Vasomotor Symptoms: 2015 Position Statement of the North American Menopause Society," *Menopause* 22, no. 11 (2015): 1155–72; quiz 1173–74.

Page 140. **antidepressants may be more helpful than HRT in specific circumstances:** David R. Rubinow, Sarah Lanier Johnson, Peter J. Schmidt, et al., "Efficacy of Estradiol in Perimenopausal Depression: So Much Promise and So Few Answers," *Depression & Anxiety Journal* 32, no. 8 (2015): 539–49.

Page 140. **Low-dose paroxetine can significantly reduce:** James A. Simon, David J. Portman, Andrew M. Kaunitz, et al., "Low-Dose Paroxetine 7.5 mg for Menopausal Vasomotor Symptoms: Two Randomized Controlled Trials," *Menopause* 20, no. 10 (2013): 1027–35.

Page 141. **Other antidepressants—citalopram:** "Nonhormonal Management of Menopause-Associated Vasomotor Symptoms: 2015 Position Statement of the North American Menopause Society."

Page 141. **desvenlafaxine was shown to reduce hot flashes by 62 percent:** JoAnn V. Pinkerton, Ginger Constantine, Eunhee Hwang, and Ru-Fong J. Cheng; Study 3353 Investigators, "Desvenlafaxine Compared with Placebo for Treatment of Menopausal Vasomotor Symptoms: A 12-Week, Multicenter, Parallel-Group, Randomized, Double-Blind, Placebo-Controlled Efficacy Trial," *Menopause* 20, no. 1 (2013): 28–37.

Page 141. **Escitalopram reduced hot flash severity by about 50 percent:** Ellen W. Freeman, Katherine A. Guthrie, Bette Caan, et al., "Efficacy of Escitalopram for Hot Flashes in Healthy Menopausal Women: A Randomized Controlled Trial," *JAMA* 305, no. 3 (2011): 267–74.

Page 142. **reduction in the frequency of moderate to severe hot flashes:** Samuel Lederman, Faith D. Ottery, Antonio Cano, et al., "Fezolinetant for Treatment of Moderate to Severe Vasomotor Symptoms Associated with Menopause (SKYLIGHT 1): A Phase 3 Randomized Controlled Study," *Lancet* 401 (2023): 1091–1102.

Page 142. **Gabapentin . . . improved the frequency and severity of hot flashes:** "Nonhormonal Management of Menopause-Associated Vasomotor Symptoms: 2015 Position Statement of the North American Menopause Society."

Page 143. **less effective than antidepressants or gabapentin:** "Nonhormonal Management of Menopause-Associated Vasomotor Symptoms: 2015 Position Statement of the North American Menopause Society."

Page 143. **Oxybutynin:** "Nonhormonal Management of Menopause-Associated Vasomotor Symptoms: 2015 Position Statement of the North American Menopause Society."

CHAPTER 11: CANCER THERAPIES AND "CHEMO BRAIN"

Page 144. **Every year, 1.4 million women worldwide are diagnosed:** Farin Kamangar, Graça M. Dores, and William F. Anderson, "Patterns of Cancer Incidence, Mortality, and Prevalence Across Five Continents: Defining Priorities to Reduce Cancer Disparities in Different Geographic Regions of the World," *Journal of Clinical Oncology* 24, no. 14 (2006): 2137–50.

Page 144. **60 to 80 percent of all cases:** Monica Arnedos, Cecile Vicier, Sherene Loi, et al., "Precision Medicine for Metastatic Breast Cancer—Limitations and Solutions," *Nature Reviews Clinical Oncology* 12, no. 12 (2015): 693–704.

Page 145. **40 percent of women taking estrogen-blocking tamoxifen:** Arnedos, Vicier, Loi, et al., "Precision Medicine for Metastatic Breast Cancer—Limitations and Solutions."

Page 146. **some genetic mutations can increase the risk of both cancers:** Ursula A. Matulonis, Anil K. Sood, Lesley Fallowfield, et al., "Ovarian Cancer," *Nature Reviews Disease Primers* 2 (2016): 16061.

Page 147. **BSO is of established benefit:** Elizabeth Casiano Evans, Kristen A. Matteson, Francisco J. Orejuela, et al., "Salpingo-Oophorectomy at the Time of Benign Hysterectomy: A Systematic Review," *Obstetrics and Gynecology* 128, no. 3 (2016): 476–85.

Page 147. **recommended in patients with significant family history:** Evans, Matteson, Orejuela, et al., "Salpingo-Oophorectomy at the Time of Benign Hysterectomy: A Systematic Review."

Page 148. **chemo brain is associated with measurable changes:** Steven Jett, Niharika Malviya, Eva Schelbaum, et al., "Endogenous and Exogenous Estrogen Exposures: How Women's Reproductive Health Can Drive Brain Aging and Inform Alzheimer's Prevention," *Frontiers in Aging Neuroscience* 14 (2022): 831807.

Page 148. **parts of the brain involved in cognitive functions:** Michiel de Ruiter, Liesbeth Reneman, Willem Boogerd, et al., "Late Effects of High-Dose Adjuvant Chemotherapy on White and Gray Matter in Breast Cancer Survivors: Converging Results from Multimodal Magnetic Resonance Imaging," *Human Brain Mapping* 33, no. 12 (2012): 2971–83.

Page 148. **chemo brain is a symptom reported:** Jeffrey S. Wefel, Shelli R. Kesler, Kyle R. Noll, and Sanne B. Schagen, "Clinical Characteristics, Pathophysiology, and Management of Noncentral Nervous System Cancer-Related Cognitive Impairment in Adults," *CA: A Cancer Journal for Clinicians* 65, no. 2 (2015): 123–38.

Page 150. **the major culprit behind the brain fog:** Wefel, Kesler, Noll, and Schagen, "Clinical Characteristics, Pathophysiology, and Management of Noncentral Nervous System Cancer-Related Cognitive Impairment in Adults."

Page 150. **negative effects on memory:** Wilbert Zwart, Huub Terra, Sabine C. Linn, and Sanne B. Schagen, "Cognitive Effects of Endocrine Therapy for Breast Cancer: Keep Calm and Carry On?," *Nature Reviews Clinical Oncology* 12, no. 10 (2015): 597–606.

Page 150. **aromatase inhibitors don't seem to have clear negative effects:** Zwart, Terra, Linn, and Schagen, "Cognitive Effects of Endocrine Therapy for Breast Cancer: Keep Calm and Carry On?"

Page 150. **patients treated with tamoxifen don't have an increased risk of dementia:** Gregory L. Branigan, Maira Soto, Leigh Neumayer, et al., "Association Between Hormone-Modulating Breast Cancer Therapies and Incidence of Neurodegenerative Outcomes for Women with Breast Cancer," *JAMA Network Open* 3 (2020): e201541–e201541.

Page 151. **Exemestane:** Branigan, Soto, Neumayer, et al., "Association Between Hormone-Modulating Breast Cancer Therapies and Incidence of Neurodegenerative Outcomes for Women with Breast Cancer."

Page 153. **lack of safety data supporting the use of systemic:** NAMS 2022 Hormone Therapy Position Statement Advisory Panel, "The 2022 Hormone Therapy Position Statement of the North American Menopause Society," *Menopause* 29, no. 7 (2022): 767–94.

Page 153. **increased risk of the cancer regrowing:** "Joint Position Statement by the British Menopause Society, Royal College of Obstetricians and Gynaecologists and Society for Endocrinology on Best Practice Recommendations for the Care of Women Experiencing the Menopause," https://www.endocrinology.org/media/d3pbn14o/joint-position-statement -on-best-practice-recommendations-for-the-care-of-women-experiencing-the -menopause.pdf.

Page 153. **the North American Menopause Society adds "in exceptional cases":** NAMS 2022 Hormone Therapy Position Statement Advisory Panel, "The 2022 Hormone Therapy Position Statement of the North American Menopause Society."

Page 153. **be offered to patients with severe menopausal symptoms:** "Joint Position Statement by the British Menopause Society, Royal College of Obstetricians and Gynaecologists, and Society for Endocrinology on Best

Practice Recommendations for the Care of Women Experiencing the Menopause."

Page 153. **"based on considerations of the many benefits of estrogen therapy":** NAMS 2022 Hormone Therapy Position Statement Advisory Panel, "The 2022 Hormone Therapy Position Statement of the North American Menopause Society."

Page 153. **low-dose vaginal estradiol and DHEA:** NAMS 2022 Hormone Therapy Position Statement Advisory Panel, "The 2022 Hormone Therapy Position Statement of the North American Menopause Society."

Page 153. **SERMS can be engineered:** Lon S. Schneider, Gerson Hernandez, Liqin Zhao, et al., "Safety and Feasibility of Estrogen Receptor-Beta Targeted PhytoSERM Formulation for Menopausal Symptoms: Phase 1b/2a Randomized Clinical Trial," *Menopause* 26 (2019): 874–84.

Page 155. **hormone therapy is viable for:** NAMS 2022 Hormone Therapy Position Statement Advisory Panel, "The 2022 Hormone Therapy Position Statement of the North American Menopause Society."

Page 155. **The same applies to mutation carriers:** Joanne Kotsopoulos, Jacek Gronwald, Beth Y. Karlan, et al., "Hormone Replacement Therapy After Oophorectomy and Breast Cancer Risk Among *BRCA1* Mutation Carriers," *JAMA Oncology* 4, no. 8 (2018): 1059–66.

CHAPTER 12: GENDER-AFFIRMING THERAPY

Page 158. **often face significant challenges in accessing appropriate healthcare:** Jaime M. Grant, Lisa A. Mottet, Justin Tanis, et al., *Injustice at Every Turn: A Report of the National Transgender Discrimination Survey* (Washington: National Center for Transgender Equality and National Gay and Lesbian Task Force, 2011).

Page 158. **lack training in transgender healthcare:** Grant, Mottet, Tanis, et al., *Injustice at Every Turn: A Report of the National Transgender Discrimination Survey.*

Page 160. **gender dysphoria:** Sam Winter, Milton Diamond, Jamison Green, et al., "Transgender People: Health at the Margins of Society," *Lancet* 388, no. 10042 (2016): 390–400.

Page 160. **being in a body that does not feel like your own:** Karen I. Fredriksen-Goldsen, Loree Cook-Daniels, Hyun-Jun Kim, et al., "Physical and Mental Health of Transgender Older Adults: An At-Risk and Underserved Population," *Gerontologist* 54, no. 3 (2014): 488–500.

Page 161. **procedures and assistance are associated with improved quality of life:** Winter, Diamond, Green, et al., "Transgender People: Health at the Margins of Society."

Page 162. **increased body hair growth, scalp hair loss, and increase in muscle mass:** Michael S. Irwig, "Testosterone Therapy for Transgender Men," *Lancet Diabetes & Endocrinology* 5, no. 4 (2017): 301–11.

Page 164. **specific brain regions of transgender women had indeed grown smaller:** Hilleke E. Hulshoff Pol, Peggy T. Cohen-Kettenis, Neeltje E. M. Van Haren, et al., "Changing Your Sex Changes Your Brain: Influences of Testosterone and Estrogen on Adult Human Brain Structure," *European Journal of Endocrinology* 155, no. 1 (2006): S107–S114.

Page 164. **specific brain regions of transgender women had indeed grown smaller:** Leire Zubiaurre-Elorza, Carme Junque, Esther Gómez-Gil, and Antonio

Guillamon, "Effects of Cross-Sex Hormone Treatment on Cortical Thickness in Transsexual Individuals," *Journal of Sexual Medicine* 11, no. 5 (2014): 1248–61.

Page 164. **their connectivity had increased:** Giancarlo Spizzirri, Fábio Luis Souza Duran, Tiffany Moukel Chaim-Avancini, et al., "Grey and White Matter Volumes Either in Treatment-Naïve or Hormone-Treated Transgender Women: A Voxel-Based Morphometry Study," *Scientific Reports* 8, no. 1 (2018): 736.

Page 164. **some of the structural characteristics of a "female" brain:** Maiko Schneider, Poli M. Spritzer, Luciano Minuzzi, et al., "Effects of Estradiol Therapy on Resting-State Functional Connectivity of Transgender Women After Gender-Affirming Related Gonadectomy," *Frontiers in Neuroscience* 13 (2019): 817.

Page 164. **treatment with testosterone and/or anti-estrogen medicines:** Pol, Cohen-Kettenis, Van Haren, et al., "Changing Your Sex Changes Your Brain: Influences of Testosterone and Estrogen on Adult Human Brain Structure"; Zubiaurre-Elorza, Junque, Gómez-Gil, and Guillamon, "Effects of Cross-Sex Hormone Treatment on Cortical Thickness in Transsexual Individuals."

Page 164. **GAT appears to align a person's brain:** Antonio Guillamon, Carme Junque, and Esther Gómez-Gil, "A Review of the Status of Brain Structure Research in Transsexualism," *Archives of Sexual Behavior* 45 (2016): 1615–48.

Page 164. **GAT changes the brain:** Ai-Min Bao and Dick F. Swaab, "Sexual Differentiation of the Human Brain: Relation to Gender Identity, Sexual Orientation and Neuropsychiatric Disorders," *Frontiers in Neuroendocrinology* 32, no. 2 (2011): 214–26.

Page 164. **transgender men receiving testosterone therapy:** Rebecca Seguin, David M. Buchner, Jingmin Liu, et al., "Sedentary Behavior and Mortality in Older Women: The Women's Health Initiative," *American Journal of Preventive Medicine* 46, no. 2 (2014): 122–35.

Page 165. **Transgender women may experience:** Bao and Swaab, "Sexual Differentiation of the Human Brain: Relation to Gender Identity, Sexual Orientation and Neuropsychiatric Disorders."

Page 165. **no clear negative effects in the short term:** Maria A. Karalexi, Marios K. Georgakis, Nikolaos G. Dimitriou, et al., "Gender-Affirming Hormone Treatment and Cognitive Function in Transgender Young Adults: A Systematic Review and Meta-Analysis," *Psychoneuroendocrinology* 119 (2020): 104721.

Page 165. **somewhat enhanced visuospatial performance:** Karalexi, Georgakis, Dimitriou, et al., "Gender-Affirming Hormone Treatment and Cognitive Function in Transgender Young Adults: A Systematic Review and Meta-Analysis."

CHAPTER 13: EXERCISE

Page 172. **a decline in your metabolic rate and lean muscle:** Natalia Grindler and Nanette F. Santoro, "Menopause and Exercise," *Menopause* 22, no. 12 (2015): 1351–58.

Page 172. **while aging *may* cause weight gain:** Grindler and Santoro, "Menopause and Exercise."

Page 172. **Midlife women tend to gain an average of 4 to 5 pounds:** Barbara Sternfeld, Hua Wang, Charles P. Quesenberry Jr., et al., "Physical Activity and Changes in Weight and Waist Circumference in Midlife Women: Findings from the Study of Women's Health Across the Nation," *American Journal of Epidemiology* 160, no. 9 (2004): 912–22.

Page 172. **increases in weight and waistline are *temporary*:** Barbara Sternfeld, Aradhana K. Bhat, Hua Wang, et al., "Menopause, Physical Activity, and Body Composition/Fat Distribution in Midlife Women," *Medicine & Science in Sports & Exercise* 37, no. 7 (2005): 1195–1202.

Page 173. **greatly improve their body composition:** Sternfeld, Bhat, Wang, et al., "Menopause, Physical Activity, and Body Composition/Fat Distribution in Midlife Women."

Page 173. **the loss of estrogen's beneficial effects:** JiWon Choi, Yolanda Guiterrez, Catherine Gilliss, and Kathryn A. Lee, "Physical Activity, Weight, and Waist Circumference in Midlife Women," *Health Care for Women International* 33, no. 2 (2012): 1086–95.

Page 173. **As little as twelve weeks of training:** Jing Zhang, Guiping Chen, Weiwei Lu, et al., "Effects of Physical Exercise on Health-Related Quality of Life and Blood Lipids in Perimenopausal Women: A Randomized Placebo-Controlled Trial," *Menopause* 21, no. 12 (2014): 1269–76.

Page 173. **promotes healthy blood pressure at all ages:** Andrés F. Loaiza-Betancur, Iván Chulvi-Medrano, Víctor A. Díaz-López, and Cinta Gómez-Tómas, "The Effect of Exercise Training on Blood Pressure in Menopause and Postmenopausal Women: A Systematic Review of Randomized Controlled Trials," *Maturitas* 149 (2021): 40–55.

Page 173. **a much lower risk of heart disease:** JoAnn E. Manson, Philip Greenland, Andrea Z. LaCroix, et al., "Walking Compared with Vigorous Exercise for the Prevention of Cardiovascular Events in Women," *New England Journal of Medicine* 347, no. 10 (2002): 716–25.

Page 174. **reductions in, and sometimes complete elimination of, hot flashes:** Candyce H. Kroenke, Bette J. Caan, Marcia L. Stefanick, et al., "Effects of a Dietary Intervention and Weight Change on Vasomotor Symptoms in the Women's Health Initiative," *Menopause* 19, no. 9 (2011): 980–88.

Page 174. **28 percent less likely to have severe hot flashes:** Juan E. Blümel, Juan Fica, Peter Chedraui, et al., "Sedentary Lifestyle in Middle-Aged Women Is Associated with Severe Menopausal Symptoms and Obesity," *Menopause* 23, no. 5 (2016): 488–93.

Page 174. **49 percent fewer hot flashes:** Janet R. Guthrie, Anthony M. A. Smith, Lorraine Dennerstein, and Carol Morse, "Physical Activity and the Menopause Experience: A Cross-Sectional Study," *Maturitas* 20, no. 2–3 (1994): 71–80.

Page 174. **a marked reduction in hot flashes in as little as three months' time:** Tom G. Bailey, N. Timothy Cable, Nabil Aziz, et al., "Exercise Training Reduces the Frequency of Menopausal Hot Flushes by Improving Thermoregulatory Control," *Menopause* 23, no. 7 (2016): 708–18.

Page 174. **awaken less during the night:** Maya J. Lambiase and Rebecca C. Thurston, "Physical Activity and Sleep Among Midlife Women with Vasomotor Symptoms," *Menopause* 20, no. 9 (2013): 946–52.

Page 174. **improved quality of sleep:** Kirsi Mansikkamäki, Jani Raitanen, Clas-Håkan Nygard, et al., "Sleep Quality and Aerobic Training Among Menopausal Women—A Randomized Controlled Trial," *Maturitas* 72, no. 4 (2012): 339–45.

Page 174. **suffer less from insomnia:** Jacobo Á Rubio-Arias, Elena Marín-Cascales, Domingo J. Ramos-Campo, et al., "Effect of Exercise on Sleep Quality and Insomnia in Middle-Aged Women: A Systematic Review and Meta-Analysis of Randomized Controlled Trials," *Maturitas* 100 (2017): 49–56.

Page 175. **a better quality of life:** Lily Stojanovska, Vasso Apostolopoulos, Remco Polman, and Erika Borkoles, "To Exercise, or, Not to Exercise, During Menopause and Beyond," *Maturitas* 77, no. 4 (2014): 318–23.

Page 175. **regular exercise significantly reduced depressive symptoms:** Faustino R. Pérez-López, Samuel J. Martínez-Domínguez, Héctor Lajusticia, Peter Chedraui, and the Health Outcomes Systematic Analyses Project, "Effects of Programmed Exercise on Depressive Symptoms in Midlife and Older Women: A Meta-Analysis of Randomized Controlled Trials," *Maturitas* 106 (2017): 38–47.

Page 175. **a 35 percent lower risk of developing dementia:** Nikolaos Scarmeas, Jose A. Luchsinger, Nicole Schupf, et al., "Physical Activity, Diet, and Risk of Alzheimer Disease," *JAMA* 302, no. 6 (2009): 627–37.

Page 175. **a whopping 30 percent lower risk of developing dementia:** Helena Hörder, Lena Johansson, XinXin Guo, et al., "Midlife Cardiovascular Fitness and Dementia: A 44-Year Longitudinal Population Study in Women," *Neurology* 90, no. 15 (2018): e1298–e1305.

Page 175. **more vigorous brain activity:** Miia Kivipelto, Francesca Mangialasche, and Tiia Ngandu, "Lifestyle Interventions to Prevent Cognitive Impairment, Dementia and Alzheimer Disease," *Nature Reviews Neurology* 14, no. 11 (2018): 653–66.

Page 176. **effectively slows bone loss after menopause:** Mahdieh Shojaa, Simon Von Stengel, Daniel Schoene, et al., "Effect of Exercise Training on Bone Mineral Density in Post-Menopausal Women: A Systematic Review and Meta-Analysis of Intervention Studies," *Frontiers in Physiology* 11 (2020): 652.

Page 176. **a significantly reduced risk of mortality:** Rebecca Seguin, David M. Buchner, Jingmin Liu, et al., "Sedentary Behavior and Mortality in Older Women: The Women's Health Initiative," *American Journal of Preventive Medicine* 46 (2014): 122–35.

Page 176. **27 percent less likely to die of heart disease:** Seguin, Buchner, Liu, et al., "Sedentary Behavior and Mortality in Older Women: The Women's Health Initiative."

Page 176. **the Nurses' Health Study:** B. Rockhill, W. C. Willett, J. E. Manson, et al., "Physical Activity and Mortality: A Prospective Study Among Women," *American Journal of Public Health* 91, no. 4 (2001): 578–83.

Page 176. **a 77 percent lower risk of respiratory death:** Rockhill, Willett, Manson, et al., "Physical Activity and Mortality: A Prospective Study Among Women."

Page 177. **particularly effective at supporting hormonal health:** Janet W. Rich-Edwards, Donna Spiegelman, Miriam Garland, et al., "Physical Activity, Body Mass Index, and Ovulatory Disorder Infertility," *Epidemiology* 13, no. 2 (2002): 184–90.

Page 178. **Regular, moderate-intensity exercise:** Hmwe Kyu, Victoria F. Bachman, Lily T. Alexander, et al., "Physical Activity and Risk of Breast Cancer, Colon Cancer, Diabetes, Ischemic Heart Disease, and Ischemic Stroke Events: Systematic Review and Dose-Response Meta-Analysis for the Global Burden of Disease Study 2013," *BMJ* 354 (2016): i3857.

Page 178. **associated with better sleep:** Seth A. Creasy, Tracy E. Crane, David O. Garcia, et al., "Higher Amounts of Sedentary Time Are Associated with

Short Sleep Duration and Poor Sleep Quality in Postmenopausal Women," *Sleep* 42, no. 7 (2019): zsz093.

Page 179. **cardio and resistance training at a moderate intensity:** Jennifer L. Copeland, Leslie A. Consitt, and Mark S. Tremblay, "Hormonal Responses to Endurance and Resistance Exercise in Females Aged 19–69 Years," *Journals of Gerontology Series A: Biological Sciences and Medical Sciences* 57, no. 4 (2002): B158–165.

Page 180. **the best regimen to foil hot flashes:** Bailey, Cable, Aziz, et al., "Exercise Training Reduces the Frequency of Menopausal Hot Flushes by Improving Thermoregulatory Control."

Page 180. **brisk walking can significantly improve your health:** Zhang, Chen, Lu, et al., "Effects of Physical Exercise on Health-Related Quality of Life and Blood Lipids in Perimenopausal Women: A Randomized Placebo-Controlled Trial."

Page 180. **brisk walking for 30 minutes three times a week:** Zhang, Chen, Lu, et al., "Effects of Physical Exercise on Health-Related Quality of Life and Blood Lipids in Perimenopausal Women: A Randomized Placebo-Controlled Trial."

Page 180. **walking slows down brain shrinkage:** Kirk I. Erickson, Michelle W. Voss, Ruchika Shaurya Prakash, et al., "Exercise Training Increases Size of Hippocampus and Improves Memory," *PNAS* 108, no. 7 (2011): 3017–22.

Page 180. **walking 6,000 or more steps per day:** Verônica Colpani, Karen Oppermann, and Poli Mara Spritzer, "Association Between Habitual Physical Activity and Lower Cardiovascular Risk in Premenopausal, Perimenopausal, and Postmenopausal Women: A Population-Based Study," *Menopause* 20, no. 5 (2013): 525–31.

Page 180. **9,000 to 10,000 steps may lower your risk of dementia:** Jennifer S. Rabin, Hannah Klein, Dylan R. Kirn, et al., "Associations of Physical Activity and Beta-Amyloid with Longitudinal Cognition and Neurodegeneration in Clinically Normal Older Adults," *JAMA Neurology* 76 (2019): 1203–10.

Page 180. **one hour of low-intensity physical activities has a favorable effect:** Stojanovska, Apostolopoulos, Polman, and Borkoles, "To Exercise, or, Not to Exercise, During Menopause and Beyond."

Page 181. **strengthening exercises are particularly effective at reducing anxiety:** Justin C. Strickland and Mark A. Smith, "The Anxiolytic Effects of Resistance Exercise," *Frontiers in Psychology* 5 (2014): 753.

Page 181. **poor balance is linked to frailty in older age:** Claudia Gil Araujo, Christina Grüne de Souza e Silva, Jari Antero Laukkanen, et al., "Successful 10-Second One-Legged Stance Performance Predicts Survival in Middle-Aged and Older Individuals," *British Journal of Sports Medicine* 56, no. 17 (2022).

Page 181. **you cannot balance on one foot for 10 seconds:** Gil Araujo, Grüne de Souza e Silva, Laukkanen, et al., "Successful 10-Second One-Legged Stance Performance Predicts Survival in Middle-Aged and Older Individuals."

CHAPTER 14: DIET AND NUTRITION

Page 185. **our brains rely on specific nutrients:** Lisa Mosconi, *Brain Food* (New York: Avery, 2018).

Page 185. **They are born with us:** Elizabeth Gould, "How Widespread Is Adult Neurogenesis in Mammals?" *Nature Reviews Neuroscience* 8, no. 6 (2007): 481–88.

Page 187. **the traditional Mediterranean diet:** Cinta Valls-Pedret, Aleix Sala-Vila, Mercè Serra-Mir, et al., "Mediterranean Diet and Age-Related Cognitive

Decline: A Randomized Clinical Trial," *JAMA Internal Medicine* 175, no. 7 (2015): 1094–103.

Page 187. **positive effects on blood pressure, cholesterol:** Ramon Estruch, Miguel Angel Martínez-González, Dolores Corella, et al., "Effects of a Mediterranean-Style Diet on Cardiovascular Risk Factors: A Randomized Trial," *Annals of Internal Medicine* 145, no. 1 (2006): 1–11.

Page 187. **blood glucose levels:** Rui Huo, Tingting Du, Y. Xu, et al., "Effects of Mediterranean-Style Diet on Glycemic Control, Weight Loss and Cardiovascular Risk Factors Among Type 2 Diabetes Individuals: A Meta-Analysis," *European Journal of Clinical Nutrition* 69, no. 11 (2014): 1200–8.

Page 187. **a 25 percent lower risk of heart attack and stroke:** Kyungwon Oh, Frank B. Hu, JoAnn E. Manson, et al., "Dietary Fat Intake and Risk of Coronary Heart Disease in Women: 20 Years of Follow-up of the Nurses' Health Study," *American Journal of Epidemiology* 161, no. 7 (2005): 672–79.

Page 187. **at least a 40 percent lower risk of developing depression:** Weiyao Yin, Marie Löf, Ruoqing Chen, et al., "Mediterranean Diet and Depression: A Population-Based Cohort Study," *International Journal of Behavioral Nutrition and Physical Activity* 18, no. 1 (2021): 153.

Page 187. *half* **the risk of breast cancer:** Estefanía Toledo, Jordi Salas-Salvadó, Carolina Donat-Vargas, et al., "Mediterranean Diet and Invasive Breast Cancer Risk Among Women at High Cardiovascular Risk in the PREDIMED Trial: A Randomized Clinical Trial," *JAMA Internal Medicine* 175 (2015): 1752–60.

Page 188. **a 20 percent** *decrease* **in hot flashes:** Gerrie-Cor M. Herber-Gast and Gita D. Mishra, "Fruit, Mediterranean-Style, and High-Fat and -Sugar Diets Are Associated with the Risk of Night Sweats and Hot Flushes in Midlife: Results from a Prospective Cohort Study," *American Journal of Clinical Nutrition* 97, no. 5 (2013): 1092–99.

Page 188. **associated with a later onset of menopause:** Yashvee Dunneram, Darren Charles Greenwood, Victoria J. Burley, and Janet E. Cade, "Dietary Intake and Age at Natural Menopause: Results from the UK Women's Cohort Study," *Journal of Epidemiology and Community Health* 72, no. 8 (2018): 733–40.

Page 189. **This combination seems to amplify the benefits:** Gal Tsaban, Anat Yaskolka Meir, Ehud Rinott, et al., "The Effect of Green Mediterranean Diet on Cardiometabolic Risk; A Randomised Controlled Trial," *Heart* (2020), doi: 10.1136/heartjnl-2020-317802.

Page 189. **the Green Mediterranean Diet seems to offer potentially higher protection:** Alon Kaplan, Hila Zelicha, Anat Yaskolka Meir, et al., "The Effect of a High-Polyphenol Mediterranean Diet (Green-MED) Combined with Physical Activity on Age-Related Brain Atrophy: The Dietary Intervention Randomized Controlled Trial Polyphenols Unprocessed Study (DIRECT PLUS)," *American Journal of Clinical Nutrition* 115, no. 5 (2022): 1270–81.

Page 190. **It facilitates the action of a molecule:** B. R. Goldin, M. N. Woods, D. L. Spiegelman, et al., "The Effect of Dietary Fat and Fiber on Serum Estrogen Concentrations in Premenopausal Women Under Controlled Dietary Conditions," *Cancer* 74, no. 3 suppl. (1994): 1125–31.

Page 190. **women treated for early stage breast cancer who consumed a high-fiber diet:** Ellen B. Gold, Shirley W. Flatt, John P. Pierce, et al., "Dietary Factors and Vasomotor Symptoms in Breast Cancer Survivors: The WHEL Study," *Menopause* 13, no. 3 (2006): 423–33.

Page 191. **one in every two Americans consumes:** Russell Knight, Christopher G. Davis, William Hahn, et al., "Livestock, Dairy, and Poultry Outlook: January 2021," http://www.ers.usda.gov/publications/pub-details/?pubid=100262.

Page 191. **women are winning that race:** Zachary J. Ward, Sara N. Bleich, Angie L. Cradock, et al., "Projected U.S. State-Level Prevalence of Adult Obesity and Severe Obesity," *New England Journal of Medicine* 381 (2019): 2440–50.

Page 192. **Women who eat plenty of these veggie heroes:** Miriam Adoyo Muga, Patrick Opiyo Owili, Chien-Yeh Hsu, et al., "Dietary Patterns, Gender, and Weight Status Among Middle-Aged and Older Adults in Taiwan: A Cross-Sectional Study," *BMC Geriatrics* 17 (2017): 268.

Page 192. **eating more fiber-rich veggies, fruits, and beans:** Candyce H. Kroenke, Bette J. Caan, Marcia L. Stefanick, et al., "Effects of a Dietary Intervention and Weight Change on Vasomotor Symptoms in the Women's Health Initiative," *Menopause* 19, no. 9 (2012): 980–88.

Page 192. **eating more leafy greens and cruciferous vegetables:** Zahra Aslani, Maryam Abshirini, Motahar Heidari-Beni, et al., "Dietary Inflammatory Index and Dietary Energy Density Are Associated with Menopausal Symptoms in Postmenopausal Women: A Cross-Sectional Study," *Menopause* 27, no. 5 (2020): 568–78.

Page 192. **50 percent lower odds of experiencing severe menopausal symptoms:** Sarah J. O. Nomura, Yi-Ting Hwang, Scarlett Lin Gomez, et al., "Dietary Intake of Soy and Cruciferous Vegetables and Treatment-Related Symptoms in Chinese-American and Non-Hispanic White Breast Cancer Survivors," *Breast Cancer Research and Treatment* 168, no. 2 (2018): 467–79.

Page 193. **fewer hot flashes and were in much better spirits:** Herber-Gast and Mishra, "Fruit, Mediterranean-Style, and High-Fat and -Sugar Diets Are Associated with the Risk of Night Sweats and Hot Flushes in Midlife: Results from a Prospective Cohort Study."

Page 193. **better cognitive performance:** Elizabeth E. Devore, Jae Hee Kang, Monique M. B. Breteler, and Francine Grodstein, "Dietary Intakes of Berries and Flavonoids in Relation to Cognitive Decline," *Annals of Neurology* 72, no. 1 (2012): 135–43.

Page 194. **markedly lower risk of heart disease:** Simin Liu, Walter C. Willett, Meir J. Stampfer, et al., "A Prospective Study of Dietary Glycemic Load, Carbohydrate Intake, and Risk of Coronary Heart Disease in US Women," *American Journal of Clinical Nutrition* 71, no. 6 (2000): 1455–61.

Page 194. **type 2 diabetes:** Matthias B. Schulze, Simin Liu, Eric B. Rimm, et al., "Glycemic Index, Glycemic Load, and Dietary Fiber Intake and Incidence of Type 2 Diabetes in Younger and Middle-Aged Women," *American Journal of Clinical Nutrition* 80, no. 2 (2004): 348–56.

Page 194. **depression:** James E. Gangwisch, Lauren Hale, Lorena Garcia, et al., "High Glycemic Index Diet as a Risk Factor for Depression: Analyses from the Women's Health Initiative," *American Journal of Clinical Nutrition* 102, no. 2 (2015): 454–63.

Page 194. **and dementia:** Martha Clare Morris, Christy C. Tangney, Yamin Wang, et al., "MIND Diet Associated with Reduced Incidence of Alzheimer's Disease," *Alzheimer's & Dementia* 11, no. 9 (2015): 1007–14.

Page 194. **not to mention better sleep:** James E. Gangwisch, Lauren Hale, Marie-Pierre St-Onge, et al., "High Glycemic Index and Glycemic Load Diets as

Risk Factors for Insomnia: Analyses from the Women's Health Initiative," *American Journal of Clinical Nutrition* 111 (2020): 429–39.

Page 195. **gut bacteria with the unique ability of metabolizing estrogen:** Song He, Hao Li, Zehui Yu, et al., "The Gut Microbiome and Sex Hormone-Related Diseases," *Frontiers in Microbiology* 12 (2021): 711137.

Page 196. **bacteria produce an enzyme called *beta-glucuronidase:*** James M. Baker, Layla Al-Nakkash, and Melissa M. Herbst-Kralovetz, "Estrogen-Gut Microbiome Axis: Physiological and Clinical Implications," *Maturitas* 103 (2017): 45–53.

Page 196. **A top-drawer gut is associated with a lower risk of obesity:** Marcus J. Claesson, Ian B. Jeffery, Susana Conde, et al., "Gut Microbiota Composition Correlates with Diet and Health in the Elderly," *Nature* 488, no. 7410 (2012): 178–84.

Page 196. **diets high in fiber and low in animal fat boast:** Claesson, Jeffery, Conde, et al., "Gut Microbiota Composition Correlates with Diet and Health in the Elderly."

Page 196. **eating processed foods *for as little as two weeks:*** Emily R. Leeming, Abigail J. Johnson, Tim D. Spector, Caroline I. Le Roy, "Effect of Diet on the Gut Microbiota: Rethinking Intervention Duration," *Nutrients* 11, no. 12 (2019): 2682.

Page 197. **similar in its chemical makeup to the estrogen made by our ovaries:** A. A. Franke, L. J. Custer, W. Wang, and C. Y. Shi, "HPLC Analysis of Isoflavonoids and Other Phenolic Agents from Foods and from Human Fluids," *Proceedings of the Society for Experimental Biology and Medicine* 217, no. 3 (1998): 263–73.

Page 198. **ability to latch on to estrogen receptors is only a thousandth of the strength of estradiol:** Valentina Echeverria, Florencia Echeverria, George E. Barreto, et al., "Estrogenic Plants: to Prevent Neurodegeneration and Memory Loss and Other Symptoms in Women After Menopause," *Frontiers in Pharmacology* 12 (2021): 644103.

Page 198. **very similar to the selective estrogen receptor modulators:** Echeverria, Echeverria, Barreto, et al., "Estrogenic Plants: to Prevent Neurodegeneration and Memory Loss and Other Symptoms in Women After Menopause."

Page 198. **phytoestrogens tend to adjust the estrogen level:** M-N. Chen, C-C. Lin, and C-F. Liu, "Efficacy of Phytoestrogens for Menopausal Symptoms: A Meta-Analysis and Systematic Review," *Climacteric* 18, no. 2 (2015): 260–69.

Page 199. **four times *less likely* to get breast cancer:** Patrizia Monteleone, Giulia Mascagni, Andrea Giannini, et al., "Symptoms of Menopause—Global Prevalence, Physiology and Implications," *Nature Reviews Endocrinology* 14, no. 4 (2018): 199–215.

Page 199. **soy is considered safe for women:** Cheryl L. Rock, Colleen Doyle, Wendy Demark-Wahnefried, et al., "Nutrition and Physical Activity Guidelines for Cancer Survivors," *CA: A Cancer Journal for Clinicians* 62, no. 4 (2012): 243–74.

Page 199. **soy does not increase the odds of breast tumor recurrence:** Sarah J. Nechuta, Bette J. Caan, Wendy Y. Chen, et al., "Soy Food Intake After Diagnosis of Breast Cancer and Survival: An In-Depth Analysis of Combined Evidence from Cohort Studies of US and Chinese Women," *American Journal of Clinical Nutrition* 96, no. 1 (2012): 123–32.

Page 199. **soy products are made of genetically modified soybeans:** USDA, "Adoption of Genetically Engineered Crops in the U.S.," https://www.ers

.usda.gov/data-products/adoption-of-genetically-engineered-crops-in-the-us/recent-trends-in-ge-adoption.aspx.

Page 200. **potentially lessens the number of hot flashes:** Oscar H. Franco, Rajiv Chowdhury, Jenna Troup, et al., "Use of Plant-Based Therapies and Menopausal Symptoms: A Systematic Review and Meta-Analysis," *JAMA* 315, no. 23 (2016): 2554–63.

Page 200. **a plant-based diet rich in soy reduced:** Neal D. Barnard, Hana Kahleova, Danielle N. Holtz, et al., "The Women's Study for the Alleviation of Vasomotor Symptoms (WAVS): A Randomized, Controlled Trial of a Plant-Based Diet and Whole Soybeans for Postmenopausal Women," *Menopause* 28, no. 10 (2021): 1150–56.

Page 201. **polyunsaturated fat supports women's health:** Oh, Hu, Manson, et al., "Dietary Fat Intake and Risk of Coronary Heart Disease in Women: 20 Years of Follow-up of the Nurses' Health Study."

Page 201. **and dementia:** Martha Clare Morris and Christine C. Tangney, "Dietary Fat Composition and Dementia Risk," *Neurobiology of Aging* 35, suppl. 2 (2014): S59–S64.

Page 201. **women who don't consume enough omega-3s:** Grace E. Giles, Caroline R. Mahoney, and Robin B. Kanarek, "Omega-3 Fatty Acids Influence Mood in Healthy and Depressed Individuals," *Nutrition Reviews* 71 (2013): 727–41.

Page 201. **as well as menopausal depression:** Marlene P. Freeman, Joseph R. Hibbeln, Michael Silver, et al., "Omega-3 Fatty Acids for Major Depressive Disorder Associated with the Menopausal Transition: A Preliminary Open Trial," *Menopause* 18, no. 3 (2011): 279–84.

Page 202. **those who frequently consumed nuts had a much lower risk:** F. B. Hu, M. J. Stampfer, J. E. Manson, et al., "Frequent Nut Consumption and Risk of Coronary Heart Disease in Women: Prospective Cohort Study," *BMJ* 317, no. 7169 (1998): 1341–45.

Page 203. **dairy butter increased LDL cholesterol significantly:** Kay-Tee Khaw, Stephen J. Sharp, Leila Finikarides, et al., "Randomised Trial of Coconut Oil, Olive Oil or Butter on Blood Lipids and Other Cardiovascular Risk Factors in Healthy Men and Women," *BMJ Open* 8, no. 3 (2018): e020167.

Page 203. **women who consumed more animal products:** Maryam S. Farvid, Eunyoung Cho, Wendy Y. Chen, et al., "Dietary Protein Sources in Early Adulthood and Breast Cancer Incidence: Prospective Cohort Study," *BMJ* 348 (2014): g3437.

Page 203. **replacing animal fat with vegetable fat:** Megan S. Rice, A. Heather Eliassen, Susan E. Hankinson, et al., "Breast Cancer Research in the Nurses' Health Studies: Exposures Across the Life Course," *American Journal of Public Health* 106 (2016): 1592–98.

Page 204. **cholesterol from food doesn't raise the cholesterol in the blood:** National Heart, Lung, and Blood Institute, "Blood Cholesterol: Causes and Risk Factors," https://www.nhlbi.nih.gov/health/blood-cholesterol/causes.

Page 209. **ultra-processed foods may well cause as many as one-third:** Thibault Fiolet, Bernard Srour, Laury Sellem, et al., "Consumption of Ultra-Processed Foods and Cancer Risk: Results from NutriNet-Santé Prospective Cohort," *BMJ* 360 (2018): k322.

Page 209. **salty snacks and processed meats in particular:** Renata Micha, Jose L. Peñalvo, Frederick Cudhea, et al., "Association Between Dietary Factors and Mortality from Heart Disease, Stroke, and Type 2 Diabetes in the United States," *JAMA* 317, no. 9 (2017): 912–24.

Page 209. **processed meat is also carcinogenic:** World Health Organization, IARC Working Group on the Evaluation of Carcinogenic Risks to Humans, *Red Meat and Processed Meat,* https://monographs.iarc.who.int/wp-content /uploads/2018/06/mono114.pdf.

Page 211. *mild* **dehydration can trigger dizziness:** Shaun K. Riebl and Brenda M. Davy, "The Hydration Equation: Update on Water Balance and Cognitive Performance," *ACSM's Health & Fitness Journal* 17, no. 6 (2013): 21–28.

Page 211. **associated with an increased risk of ovulatory infertility:** Elizabeth E. Hatch, Lauren A. Wise, Ellen M. Mikkelsen, et al., "Caffeinated Beverage and Soda Consumption and Time to Pregnancy," *Epidemiology* 23, no. 3 (2012): 393–401.

Page 212. **This may help shed pounds and stabilize weight more efficiently:** Chanthawat Patikorn, Kiera Roubal, Sajeesh K. Veettil, et al., "Intermittent Fasting and Obesity-Related Health Outcomes: An Umbrella Review of Meta-Analyses of Randomized Clinical Trials," *JAMA Network Open* 4, no. 12 (2021): e2139558.

Page 212. **health benefits of intermittent fasting** *in humans:* Rafael de Cabo and Mark P. Mattson, "Effects of Intermittent Fasting on Health, Aging, and Disease," *New England Journal of Medicine* 381 (2019): 2541–51.

CHAPTER 15: SUPPLEMENTS AND BOTANICALS

Page 215. **up to half of all women in industrialized countries:** Paul Posadzki, Myeong Soo Lee, T. W. Moon, et al., "Prevalence of Complementary and Alternative Medicine (CAM) Use by Menopausal Women: A Systematic Review of Surveys," *Maturitas* 75, no. 1 (2013): 34–43.

Page 216. **phytoestrogen supplements:** P. A. Komesaroff, C. V. Black, V. Cable, and K. Sudhir, "Effects of Wild Yam Extract on Menopausal Symptoms, Lipids and Sex Hormones in Healthy Menopausal Women," *Climacteric* 4, no. 2 (2001): 144–50.

Page 217. **about half reporting decreases in hot flashes:** Oscar H. Franco, Rajiv Chowdhury, Jenna Troup, et al., "Use of Plant-Based Therapies and Menopausal Symptoms: A Systematic Review and Meta-Analysis," *JAMA* 315, no. 23 (2016): 2554–63.

Page 217. **soothing mild to moderate night sweats:** Francesca Borrelli and Edzard Ernst, "Alternative and Complementary Therapies for the Menopause," *Maturitas* 66, no. 4 (2010): 333–43.

Page 217. **black cohosh doesn't appear to have estrogenic effects:** Wolfgang Wuttke, Hubertus Jarry, Jutta Haunschild, et al., "The Non-Estrogenic Alternative for the Treatment of Climacteric Complaints: Black Cohosh (Cimicifuga or Actaea racemosa)," *Journal of Steroid Biochemistry and Molecular Biology* 139 (2014): 302–10.

Page 217. **chaste tree berry seems to have hormone-balancing effects:** Franco, Chowdhury, Troup, et al., "Use of Plant-Based Therapies and Menopausal Symptoms: A Systematic Review and Meta-Analysis."

Page 218. **clinical trials to date have not shown effects on hot flashes:** Franco, Chowdhury, Troup, et al., "Use of Plant-Based Therapies and Menopausal Symptoms: A Systematic Review and Meta-Analysis."

Page 218. **this oil is often recommended for treating hot flashes:** R. Chenoy, S. Hussain, Y. Tayob, et al., "Effect of Oral Gamolenic Acid from Evening Primrose Oil on Menopausal Flushing," *BMJ* 308, no. 6927 (1994): 501–503.

Page 218. **may help with breast tenderness:** Sandhya Pruthi, Dietlind L. Wahner-Roedler, Carolyn J. Torkelson, et al., "Vitamin E and Evening Primrose Oil for Management of Cyclical Mastalgia: A Randomized Pilot Study," *Alternative Medicine Review* 15, no. 1 (2010): 59–67.

Page 219. **ginseng can improve symptoms of menopausal depression:** Myung-Sunny Kim, Hyun-Ja Lim, Hye Jeong Yang, et al., "Ginseng for Managing Menopause Symptoms: A Systematic Review of Randomized Clinical Trials," *Journal of Ginseng Research* 37, no. 1 (2013): 30–36.

Page 219. **ginseng doesn't consistently help with vasomotor symptoms:** Franco, Chowdhury, Troup, et al., "Use of Plant-Based Therapies and Menopausal Symptoms: A Systematic Review and Meta-Analysis."

Page 220. **phytoestrogens decrease the number and frequency of hot flashes:** Franco, Chowdhury, Troup, et al., "Use of Plant-Based Therapies and Menopausal Symptoms: A Systematic Review and Meta-Analysis."

Page 220. **some soy isoflavones:** Franco, Chowdhury, Troup, et al., "Use of Plant-Based Therapies and Menopausal Symptoms: A Systematic Review and Meta-Analysis."

Page 220. **a 50 percent reduction in hot flashes:** Alessandra Crisafulli, Herbert Marini, Alessandra Bitto, et al., "Effects of Genistein on Hot Flushes in Early Postmenopausal Women: A Randomized, Double-Blind EPT- and Placebo-Controlled Study," *Menopause* 11, no. 4 (2004): 400–404.

Page 220. **positive effects on bone mineral density:** De-Fu Ma, Lin-Qiang Qin, Pei-Yu Wang, and Ryohei Katoh, "Soy Isoflavone Intake Increases Bone Mineral Density in the Spine of Menopausal Women: Meta-Analysis of Randomized Controlled Trials," *Clinical Nutrition* 27, no. 1 (2008): 57–64.

Page 220. **soy effects vary according to genetic background:** Kenneth D. R. Setchell, Nadine M. Brown, Linda Zimmer-Nechemias, et al., "Evidence for Lack of Absorption of Soy Isoflavone Glycosides in Humans, Supporting the Crucial Role of Intestinal Metabolism for Bioavailability," *American Journal of Clinical Nutrition* 76, no. 2 (2002): 447–53.

Page 221. **red clover isoflavones taken for ninety days:** Marcus Lipovac, Peter Chedraui, Christine Gruenhut, et al., "The Effect of Red Clover Isoflavone Supplementation over Vasomotor and Menopausal Symptoms in Postmenopausal Women," *Gynecological Endocrinology* 28, no. 3 (2012): 203–207.

Page 221. **no evidence that flaxseed helps with hot flashes:** An Pan, Danxia Yu, Wendy Demark-Wahnefried, et al., "Meta-Analysis of the Effects of Flaxseed Interventions on Blood Lipids," *American Journal of Clinical Nutrition* 90, no. 2 (2009): 288–97.

Page 222. **rhodiola may help balance the stress hormone cortisol:** V. Darbinyan, A. Kteyan, A. Panossian, et al., "Rhodiola Rosea in Stress Induced Fatigue—A Double Blind Cross-Over Study of a Standardized Extract SHR-5 with a Repeated Low-Dose Regimen on the Mental Performance of Healthy Physicians During Night Duty," *Phytomedicine* 7, no. 5 (2000): 365–71.

Page 222. **St. John's wort is effective for mild to moderate anxiety:** Klaus Linde, Michael Berner, Matthias Egger, and Cynthia Mulrow, "St John's Wort for Depression: Meta-Analysis of Randomised Controlled Trials," *British Journal of Psychiatry* 186 (2005): 99–107.

Page 222. **some professional societies consider St. John's wort a viable option:** Franco, Chowdhury, Troup, et al., "Use of Plant-Based Therapies and Menopausal Symptoms: A Systematic Review and Meta-Analysis."

Page 223. **to energize and improve sexual function in men:** Wenyi Zhu, Yijie Du, Hong Meng, et al., "A Review of Traditional Pharmacological Uses, Phytochemistry, and Pharmacological Activities of *Tribulus terrestris*," *Chemistry Central Journal* J 11, no. 1 (2017): 60.

Page 223. **improve the sleep quality in postmenopausal women:** C. Stevinson and E. Ernst, "Valerian for Insomnia: A Systematic Review of Randomized Clinical Trials," *Sleep Medicine* 1, no. 2 (2000): 91–99.

Page 223. **B vitamins may help reduce stress:** Nahid Yazdanpanah, M. Carola Zillikens, Fernando Rivadeneira, et al., "Effect of Dietary B Vitamins on BMD and Risk of Fracture in Elderly Men and Women: The Rotterdam Study," *Bone* 41, no. 6 (2007): 987–94.

Page 225. **the effects of magnesium supplements on sleep:** Jasmine Mah and Tyler Pitre, "Oral Magnesium Supplementation for Insomnia in Older Adults: A Systematic Review & Meta-Analysis," *BMC Complementary Medicine and Therapies* 21, no. 1 (2021): 125.

Page 225. **omega-3 supplements may help reduce night sweats:** Mina Mohammady, Leila Janani, Shayesteh Jahanfar, and Mahsa Sadat Mousavi, "Effect of Omega-3 Supplements on Vasomotor Symptoms in Menopausal Women: A Systematic Review and Meta-Analysis," *European Journal of Obstetrics & Gynecology and Reproductive Biology* 228 (2018): 295–302.

Page 225. **depressed mood associated with menopause:** Yuhua Liao, Bo Xie, Huimin Zhang, et al., "Efficacy of Omega-3 PUFAs in Depression: A Meta-Analysis," *Translational Psychiatry* 9, no. 1 (2019): 190.

Page 226. **fewer hot flashes after four weeks of vitamin E supplementation:** Alisa Johnson, Lynae Roberts, and Gary Elkins, "Complementary and Alternative Medicine for Menopause," *Journal of Evidence-Based Integrative Medicine* 24 (2019): 2515690X19829380.

Page 226. **a 35 to 40 percent reduction in hot flashes:** D. L. Barton, C. L. Loprinzi, S. K. Quella, et al., "Prospective Evaluation of Vitamin E for Hot Flashes in Breast Cancer Survivors," *Journal of Clinical Oncology* 16, no. 2 (1998): 495–500.

CHAPTER 16: STRESS REDUCTION AND SLEEP HYGIENE

Page 227. **women report considerably higher stress levels:** American Psychological Association, "Stress in America Findings," November 9, 2010, https://www .apa.org/news/press/releases/stress/2010/national-report.pdf.

Page 229. **lowering your ability to recover from common colds:** E. Ron de Kloet, Marian Joëls, and Florian Holsboer, "Stress and the Brain: From Adaptation to Disease," *Nature Reviews Neuroscience* 6, no. 6 (2005): 463–75.

Page 229. **a high-stress life might mean memory loss:** Justin B. Echouffo-Tcheugui, Sarah C. Conner, Jayandra J. Himali, et al., "Circulating Cortisol and Cognitive and Structural Brain Measures: The Framingham Heart Study," *Neurology* 91, no. 21 (2018): e1961–e1970.

Page 230. **practicing yoga for at least twelve weeks positively affects:** Holger Cramer, Romy Lauche, Jost Langhorst, and Gustav Dobos, "Effectiveness of Yoga for Menopausal Symptoms: A Systematic Review and Meta-Analysis of Randomized Controlled Trials," *Evidence-Based Complementary and Alternative Medicine* 2012 (2012): 863905.

Page 231. **women who practice yoga also tend to have reduced symptoms of stress:** Katherine M. Newton, Susan D. Reed, Katherine A. Guthrie, et al., "Efficacy of Yoga for Vasomotor Symptoms: A Randomized Controlled Trial," *Menopause* 21, no. 4 (2014): 339–46.

Page 231. **an improved physical quality of life:** Thi Mai Nguyen, Thi Thanh Toan Do, Tho Nhi Tran, and Jin Hee Kim, "Exercise and Quality of Life in Women with Menopausal Symptoms: A Systematic Review and Meta-Analysis of Randomized Controlled Trials," *International Journal of Environmental Research and Public Health* 17, no. 19 (2020): 7049.

Page 231. **the power to protect us from stress overload:** Madhav Goyal, Sonal Singh, Erica M. S. Sibinga, et al., "Meditation Programs for Psychological Stress and Well-Being: A Systematic Review and Meta-Analysis," *JAMA Internal Medicine* 174, no. 3 (2014): 357–68.

Page 231. **MBSR led to meaningful improvements in overall quality of life:** James Francis Carmody, Sybil Crawford, Elena Salmoirago-Blotcher, et al., "Mindfulness Training for Coping with Hot Flashes: Results of a Randomized Trial," *Menopause* 18, no. 6 (2011): 611–20.

Page 231. **MBSR and cognitive therapy was just as effective:** Zindel V. Segal, Peter Bieling, Trevor Young, et al., "Antidepressant Monotherapy vs Sequential Pharmacotherapy and Mindfulness-Based Cognitive Therapy, or Placebo, for Relapse Prophylaxis in Recurrent Depression," *Archives of General Psychiatry* 67, no. 12 (2010): 1256–64.

Page 231. **shown to reduce inflammation while improving memory, sleep, and mental clarity:** Dharma Singh Khalsa, "Stress, Meditation, and Alzheimer's Disease Prevention: Where the Evidence Stands," *Journal of Alzheimer's Disease* 48 (2015): 1–12.

Page 232. **can reduce hot flashes and poses little risk:** "Nonhormonal Management of Menopause-Associated Vasomotor Symptoms: 2015 Position Statement of the North American Menopause Society," *Menopause* 22, no. 11 (2015): 1155–72; quiz 1173–74.

Page 233. **69 percent reduction in hot flash severity:** Alisa Johnson, Lynae Roberts, and Gary Elkins, "Complementary and Alternative Medicine for Menopause," *Journal of Evidence-Based Integrative Medicine* 24 (2019): 2515690X19829380.

Page 233. **hypnosis also reduced hot flashes by 50 to 74 percent:** Gary R. Elkins, William I. Fisher, Aimee K. Johnson, et al., "Clinical Hypnosis in the Treatment of Postmenopausal Hot Flashes: A Randomized Controlled Trial," *Menopause* 20, no. 3 (2013): 291–98.

Page 233. **CBT is recommended by the North American Menopause Society:** "Nonhormonal Management of Menopause-Associated Vasomotor Symptoms: 2015 Position Statement of the North American Menopause Society."

Page 235. **oxytocin may be behind women's unique impulse to tend and befriend:** S. E. Taylor, L. C. Klein, B. P. Lewis, et al., "Biobehavioral Responses to Stress in Females: Tend-and-Befriend, Not Fight-or-Flight," *Psychological Review* 107, no. 3 (2000): 411–29.

CHAPTER 17: TOXINS AND ESTROGEN DISRUPTERS

Page 242. **100,000 new chemicals have been released:** World Health Organization, *State of the Science of Endocrine Disrupting Chemicals 2012,* June 6, 2012, https://www.who.int/publications/i/item/9789241505031.

Page 242. **800 chemicals are either known or suspected to negatively impact our health:** World Health Organization, *State of the Science of Endocrine Disrupting Chemicals 2012.*

Page 242. **they trigger hormonal imbalances:** World Health Organization, *State of the Science of Endocrine Disrupting Chemicals 2012*.

Page 242. **hundreds of these chemicals are also toxic to *your* brain:** P. Grandjean and P. J. Landrigan, "Developmental Neurotoxicity of Industrial Chemicals," *Lancet* 368, no. 9553 (2006): P2167–P2178.

Page 242. **air pollution has become both an acknowledged health hazard:** Gill Livingston, Jonathan Huntley, Andrew Sommerlad, et al., "Dementia Prevention, Intervention, and Care: 2020 Report of the Lancet Commission," *Lancet* 396, no. 10248 (2020): 413–46.

Page 242. **xenoestrogens can do significant toxic harm to children and women:** Evanthia Diamanti-Kandarakis, Jean-Pierre Bourguignon, Linda C. Giudice, et al., "Endocrine-Disrupting Chemicals: An Endocrine Society Scientific Statement," *Endocrine Reviews* 30, no. 4 (2009): 293–42.

Page 243. **limiting exposure to environmental pollutants and chemicals:** American Academy of Pediatrics Policy Statement, "Food Additives and Child Health," *Pediatrics* 142, no. 2 (2018): e20181408.

Page 243. **accumulate these toxins at even higher levels:** Ioannis Manisalidis, Elisavet Stavropoulou, Agathangelos Stavropoulos, and Eugenia Bezirtzoglou, "Environmental and Health Impacts of Air Pollution: A Review," *Frontiers in Public Health* 8 (2020): 14.

Page 245. **more people die from smoking cigarettes:** Manisalidis, Stavropoulou, Stavropoulos, and Bezirtzoglou, "Environmental and Health Impacts of Air Pollution: A Review."

Page 245. **88 million *nonsmokers*:** "Vital Signs: Disparities in Nonsmokers' Exposure to Secondhand Smoke—United States, 1999–2012," *Morbidity and Mortality Weekly Report* 64 (2015): 103–108. See also https://www.cdc.gov/tobacco/data_statistics/fact_sheets/adult_data/cig_smoking/index.htm.

Page 245. **a significantly higher risk of painful menstrual cycles and infertility:** A. Hyland, K. Piazza, K. M. Hovey, et al., "Associations Between Lifetime Tobacco Exposure with Infertility and Age at Natural Menopause: The Women's Health Initiative Observational Study," *Tobacco Control* 25, no. 6 (2016): 706–14.

Page 245. **Hot flashes, anxiety, mood swings, and insomnia are all the more intense:** Ellen B. Gold, Alicia Colvin, Nancy Avis, et al., "Longitudinal Analysis of the Association Between Vasomotor Symptoms and Race/Ethnicity Across the Menopausal Transition: Study of Women's Health Across the Nation," *American Journal of Public Health* 96, no. 7 (2006): 1226–35.

Page 245. **Women who smoke 100 cigarettes:** Hyland, Piazza, Hovey, et al., "Associations Between Lifetime Tobacco Exposure with Infertility and Age at Natural Menopause: The Women's Health Initiative Observational Study."

CHAPTER 18: THE POWER OF A POSITIVE MINDSET

Page 254. **in societies where age is revered:** Mary Jane Minkin, "Menopause: Hormones, Lifestyle, and Optimizing Aging," *Obstetrics and Gynecology Clinics of North America* 46, no. 3 (2019): 501–14.

Page 254. **25 percent of Japanese women reportedly experience hot flashes:** J. A. Winterich and D. Umberson, "How Women Experience Menopause: The Importance of Social Context," *Journal of Women and Aging* 11, no. 4 (1999): 57–73.

Page 255. **Shoulder stiffness and frozen shoulders are:** Winterich and Umberson, "How Women Experience Menopause: The Importance of Social Context."

Page 255. **a decrease in vision:** Melissa K. Melby, Debra Anderson, Lynette Leidy Sievert, and Carla Makhlouf Obermeye, "Methods Used in Cross-Cultural Comparisons of Vasomotor Symptoms and Their Determinants," *Maturitas* 70, no. 2 (2011): 110–19.

Page 256. **a positive outlook on life in general:** Susanne Wurm, Manfred Diehl, Anna E. Kornadt, et al., "How Do Views on Aging Affect Health Outcomes in Adulthood and Late Life? Explanations for an Established Connection," *Developmental Review* 46 (2017): 27–43.

Page 256. **link between a woman's physical symptoms, her beliefs about menopause, and her actual experience:** Beverley Ayers, Mark Forshaw, and Myra S. Hunter, "The Impact of Attitudes Towards the Menopause on Women's Symptom Experience: A Systematic Review," *Maturitas* 65, no. 1 (2010): 28–36.

Page 256. **more apprehension about menopause:** Ayers, Forshaw, and Hunter, "The Impact of Attitudes Towards the Menopause on Women's Symptom Experience: A Systematic Review."

Page 256. **due to variations in psychological or emotional well-being:** Amanda A. Deeks, "Psychological Aspects of Menopause Management," *Best Practice & Research Clinical Endocrinology & Metabolism* 17, no. 1 (2003): 17–31.

Page 258. **we can change our entire philosophy about menopause:** David S. Yeager, Paul Hanselman, Gregory M. Walton, et al., "A National Experiment Reveals Where a Growth Mindset Improves Achievement," *Nature* 573, no. 7774 (2019): 364–69.

Page 259. **core curriculum for performance enhancement programs in sports:** Antonis Hatzigeorgiadis, Nikos Zourbanos, Evangelos Galanis, and Yiannis Theodorakis, "Self-Talk and Sports Performance: A Meta-Analysis," *Perspectives on Psychological Science* 6, no. 4 (2011): 348–56.

Page 259. **the heart of most psychological and mindfulness-based therapies:** Farid Chakhssi, Jannis T. Kraiss, Marion Sommers-Spijkerman, and Ernst Bohlmeijer, "The Effect of Positive Psychology Interventions on Well-Being and Distress in Clinical Samples with Psychiatric or Somatic Disorders: A Systematic Review and Meta-Analysis," *BMC Psychiatry* 18, no. 1 (2018): 211.

Page 261. **chemical bonuses in the body that can reduce stress and increase pain tolerance:** Dexter Louie, Karolina Brook, and Elizabeth Frates, "The Laughter Prescription: A Tool for Lifestyle Medicine," *American Journal of Lifestyle Medicine* 10, no. 4 (2016): 262–67.

INDEX

Note: *Italicized* page numbers indicate material in tables or illustrations.